PTSD AND ME

PTSD AND ME

PTSD AND ME

THE STORY OF MY STRUGGLE
WITH MYSELF AFTER IRAQ

RETIRED MSG DENNIS JAMES WILLIAMS

iUniverse LLC
Bloomington

PTSD and Me
The Story of My Struggle with Myself after Iraq

iUniverse books may be ordered through booksellers or by contacting:

iUniverse LLC
1663 Liberty Drive
Bloomington, IN 47403
www.iuniverse.com
1-800-Authors (1-800-288-4677)

ISBN: 978-1-4917-0020-4 (sc)
ISBN: 978-1-4917-0019-8 (hc)
ISBN: 978-1-4917-0018-1 (ebk)

Library of Congress Control Number: 2013913690

Printed in the United States of America

iUniverse rev. date: 08/05/2013

Table of Contents

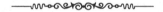

In Loving Memory of
Vladimir E. Williams
December 18, 1978 - April 20, 2013

"A Beautiful Life"

A beautiful life
that came to an end,
he died as he lived,
everyone's friend.
In our hearts a memory will
always be kept, of one we loved,
and will never forget.

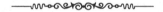

DEDICATION

THIS BOOK IS DEDICATE
TO EVERY MILITARY PERSON
WHO MAKES IT BACK TO THE STATES
BUT WHO NEVER REALLY MAKE IT HOME
I KNOW IT IS HARD
BUT YOU ARE NOT ALONE

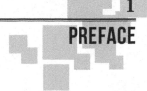

PREFACE

THIS IS NOT A SELF help book and is not intended as a substitute for the medical advice of physicians. The reader should consult a physician in matters relating to his or her health. Although I believe that one can get a good understanding of some of the PTSD issue that I had to deal with it is in no means an educated solution to them.

This book is the story of how I handled PTSD. Or one might say how PTSD handled me. The fact that I had to hit rock bottom before I finally saw what I was doing not only to myself but also to those around me. I call it the full circle that a lot of former combat veterans go through. The anger, and frustration that I felt and how I tried to manage it with out really accepting the fact that I was not myself anymore.

I invite you to read and try to understand how lost I really was. Maybe you can have a good laugh or cry at my actions. It is a journey that I don't wish on anyone yet I know that many more will experience it. Whether you are a veteran or you know someone who is one, I believe that there are signs that one can pick up on. Of course just like that alcoholic accepting that there is a problem is usually the biggest hurdle of all.

Keep the faith in tomorrow and in finding what one needs to fit in again, and remember that it is ok to ask for help when you are down or at your wits end. If you got no one you feel you can talk to talk to a stranger, or better yet call 911 the life you save just might be your own, or someone close to you.

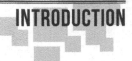
"IF IT LOOKS LIKE A DUCK
AND ACTS LIKE A DUCK,
AND SOUNDS LIKE A DUCK,
THEN BELIEVE IT OR NOT
IT IS A DUCK!'

I AM A RETIRED DISABLED combat veteran who achieved the rank of MSG / E8 in my 24 years of service to my country. I joined the U.S. Army on the delayed entry program when I was still a senior in high school and left two weeks after I graduated for basic training. All I wanted to do was to jump out of airplanes and find myself. My recruiter told me I qualified for a two year enlistment but if I wanted to go airborne that I would have to go three years. My response was that if I did not get airborne I did not want to join. He came back with if you are going to do three years you might as well do four years and get a five thousand dollar bonus when you graduate from basic training. Sure I said and not knowing or caring about any other thing then jumping out of airplanes found myself assigned to the 1/75 Airborne Infantry Ranger BN.

Basic was at Fort Benning, Georgia, and was an excited time for me. It seemed that everyday we did something different and challenging. My body was not as excited as my mind was but the drill sergeants had their ways of helping me out in this area. I was one of the few that actually gained weight in basic. Sure I had my struggles just like anyone and sure I did my share of the eight count push-up or worse the dieing cockroach, but it was what I wanted and what I needed to find myself.

Airborne school was right after basic where we had four weeks of more strenuous physical training. They taught us how to do a PLF (parachutes landing fall), which was more on how to use your entire body to absorb the impact of your landing so you had less chances of getting hurt. The hardest thing here was getting used to jumping out the door of a plane in good form. For this they had the 34 foot towers, which were 34 feet in the air and you actually jumped out but you were attached to a wire that gave the impression of jumping out of the plane and gave you enough time to count your four seconds before you checked your chute. I remember it well because I was scared and I did it all wrong till it finally sunk in that it was actually fun. Of course then instructors told me I was done now that I was just having fun.

After graduating from airborne school I was assigned to the Rangers. I wish I could say that I made this place my home but it would be a lie. My foot got infected and I was a "Ranger" so I just drove on with training till I could not put my boot on. By then the infection had grown into gang green and I had to have a chuck cut out. I was on a physical profile for too long of a time so I was reassigned to the 82nd Airborne. During my time here I was deployed in "Operation Urgent Fury" to the country of Grenada. Though my unit was only on the island a couple weeks it was one of the biggest changes in life that I went through. Not only was it such a wonderful feeling to help others and hear and see their praises and gratitude it was also the time when I no longer wondered what I would do in the face of danger and knew that I could stand and face anything that was thrown at me. It made me a better soldier deep inside of my soul. It is hard to explain but I felt whole.

Soon after coming back to Fort Bragg from Grenada, I was in the process of putting a 4187 (personnel action) form to request to go back to the Rangers when a friend of mine who was levied from Fort Bragg to Germany asked me to come over there instead. So I put on the 4187 a request to go right to his unit and it was improved. Germany was a story all in its own both on the military side as well as what we did on our free time there. From the beer to the traveling it was wonderful.

After my tour was done I decided to not re-enlist and went home, but I joined the National Guards as soon as I got there and served until I retired. I was going to retire as soon as I got my twenty years in but 9/11 came just before that and I could not see myself getting out of the military after that. Since 9/11 I have helped with the set up of security around the nuclear power plants in Oswego, was in charge of terminal 1,2,&3 of JFK Airport in NYC for six months, spent a month guarding the subways of NYC, as well as being deployed numerous times before 9/11 on the ice storm and other state emergencies.

My last deployment was to the country of Iraq with the 2/108 Infantry of the New York State National Guards, and served as the S2 NCOIC. I don't see myself as a hero just a soldier that did what I had to do when I had to do it. I don't questioned the choices that I made but I do live with the outcome of many decisions that I made.

I chose to break everything up into little organized areas. You need to try and remember that many things happened at the same time in some kind of degree. Although certain things are focus points for me, where decisions or realization of some sort finally hits home and sinks in.

Names have been deleted and changed not to protect the innocent, but to hinder any law action that one might attempt to do against me. Whether someone either can't handle the truth or they feel insulted or ashamed of what they have done or have not done. I am writing as I believe things have happened. Of course I only have my side of the story to write. If I had their side then I don't think there would have been a reason to write this book. Maybe I would not have had all the issues or fallen as far as I fell.

I will even go as far as to say that I became quick to point a finger at someone other then myself. Maybe being on edge worn me down. This book is my screaming at them and the world that I am someone! Like that little dust speck in "Horton Hears a Who". I am here. I am here!

Because this book is me standing up and fighting for who I was, or for who I became I want to dedicate this book to all the military persons who make it back to the states but who have not made it back home, whether it is in their minds or in their hearts. Maybe my struggles and actions can help them. Maybe this book will scream to them that they do matter, and no matter how hard you find it to fit in with society, or work you have to be strong and take that first step, and don't give up. You are not alone. You do have a choice.

If you are at the end of your rope and you feel you can't make it another minute,

I urge you to call 911.

Find what ever reason there is
to make it to another day.

DREAMS OR REALITY

Dreams:

- Series of thoughts, images, or emotions occurring during sleep.
- An experience of waking life having the characteristics of a dream as a visionary creation of the imagination.
- A state of mind marked by abstraction or release from reality.
- An object seen in a dreamlike state: vision.
- Something notable for its beauty, excellence, or enjoyable quality.
- A strongly desired goal or purpose.
- Something that fully satisfies a wish.

Reality:

- The quality or state of being real.
- A real event, entity or state of affairs.
- The totality of real things and events.
- Something that is neither derivative nor dependent but exists necessarily.
- In actual fact.

IT WAS JUST AN AVERAGE miserable morning. The temperature was already above 100 degrees and rising fast. The eastwardly wind had a mild breeze which only brought the stench of the surroundings to the senses and did little to cool any of the soldiers loading up in their vehicles for a mission.

The convoy was rolling out to a area that was well know to the BN (battalion). Numerous times the BN had sent out patrols that were met by IED's (improvised exploding devices) in this area. Our informant had narrowed down all of the activity to a small block. The mission to secure the area and search for materials used in the manufacturing of IED's and the detention of any and all male occupants.

My HUMVEE was just a regular cargo which had the doors taken off much to the displeasure of my BN CSM (command sergeant major). He felt it was unsafe to drive around without a door. How much protection can a plastic door really be? All it was to me was a hindrance in getting in and out of the vehicle and also made it almost impossible to fire as you were driving. But with the doors off and my M4 strapped to my vest I easily could fire with some degree of accurately as I am a left handed firer.

As we approach the target area I get an uneasy feeling. I could see no dogs, no cows. It's just too quiet. Where are all the kids that are normally running after us begging for anything and everything? Something was just not right.

All of a sudden there is a loud blast and you hear the distinct sound of AK fire followed by the musical sound of the M2 machine gun, and M4's firing back. I scan the area directly in front and to the side of me. I get a quick glimpse of movement in the small rise about 100 meters away. I suddenly see a figure standing with what appears to be a RPG (rocket propelled grenade) on his shoulder aiming right at us.

The noise and confusion is all around us. I see the flames from the RPG and I quickly scream incoming jumping out of my vehicle (so much for wanting that plastic door), and try to take cover and roll over the edge of the road into a small ditch. I try to take up a good hasty position and fire in the direction of where the RPG came from. Suddenly I feel the earth move as the RPG takes a direct hit to the vehicle directly behind mine. The M2 falls silent and for a very short period of times it seems to be all quiet. Then I realize that it was a direct hit to the vehicle and we have soldiers hurt. I hear someone in the truck moaning for help. I don't see anyone else around. Without thinking I get to my feet and turn and start to run toward the call for help.

It feels like slow motion as I attempt to make the short 20 yards to the vehicle. All of a sudden I am not running but flying through the air. All I can hear is my ears ringing. I am thrown off the road and down a little slope. My M4 is gone and I am dazed. I hear voices and it is not English but Arabic. I feel a firm grip on my left shoulder. With all the strength that I have left I lash out and swing my right fist over my left shoulder and make a direct contact with the face of the Iraqi who has grabbed me. I hear the moan and see the blood start to come from their nose. I feel their grasp lighten but I am not free yet. I let out a loud piercing yell to alert my fellow soldiers that I am in trouble.

Suddenly I bolt upright, and look around, dazed and confused and with a blurry grey view. Slowly reality starts to take hold and I remember where I am and wonder what happened to the person that

I just swung at. For a brief moment I am confused and unsure about where I am or what is going on. I don't dare move and I freeze like a deer at night being shined by a spotlight. My vision starts to clear and I see my wife's face come into focus and I see the blood running out of her nose. Still I sit there wondering what is real and what a nightmare is as I try to focus on what is happening in my mind. I can't seem to calm down or even relax. I know that the chances of me even closing my eyes again are over for the night.

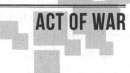

THE ACT OF WAR SEEMS like it would be hard to some. Especially to those who have never served in the armed forces. The truth is war is simple and easy for the most part; you just concentrate on the now. Weapons, ammunition, men, mission, sleep chow, mission, buddies, staying alert, and now and then you throw in a shower. With all the training you get to the point where you are almost a robot reacting to what goes on around you. You follow your orders and missions and try to stay focused. The memories of the life you left behind seem so far away and can get more distance with time, and situations that go on. Your programming instills in you the reaction time for indirect fires, reaction to contact, and the dreaded IED going off. You do your job simple put. You do your job because that is who you are now. To think of the home life leaves you less focused. Most people who have loved ones in harms way always worry when they hear nothing from them. The truth is that no news is good news. If something bad was to happen to you your family would be the first to know. For they lock all phones and computers down until the next of kin is notified. Nothing can be worse than hearing on the news that your loved one whether it is a solider or a civilian contractor is hurt or worse dead.

What the
Army
Requires of you

War:
- Armed conflict between nations, states, or factions.
- A determined struggle especially for a specific goal
- A state of antagonism or discord
- Military techniques or procedures as a science
  - To engage in armed conflict
  - To struggle or contend

Working
Around
Reality

W.A.R. (working around reality). I would have to say the first step here is to figure out what is reality and what is a fantasy or what is the realty in someone's brain. If you believe the reality in your brain over what others perceive to be reality, then is it not reality to you? What a question to ask the doctors out there. Is it better to make someone believe that reality is better than what one might believe to be reality? I guess the human in us says to ourselves that we need to make someone see the same as we see things. I bet many debates could be given over this. It is my belief that the effort should be made to make someone see the real reality and to get away from what someone perceives to be their reality.

If you act or react to a thought or a feeling, is this not real. Is it not real at least to you? I would have to say that what I thought or felt was true was a little tainted to say the least. It seemed the more I thought that things were a certain way the more they were that way. It is sort of like a catch 22. How do we change that thought, and the better question how do we get to the point where we know that we need to do something to change things? I bet there is some out there who are copping but who are on the edge in ways. Maybe this is where we get the POSTAL SYDROM from.

I guess it is a little like being an alcoholic. When does it get to the point where the alcohol is controlling you? The better question is how we know that it is controlling us. Surely no one wants to admit that they have fallen prey to something that "normal" people do every day. How do we get someone to sit and really think about some of the choices that they have made? How can we put their decisions in front of them so bluntly that they can finally see what they have become or have given up on or worse just plain forgot about? For I know that the sanctuary that I built up to protect myself can and did turn into a prison. The key was finally realizing that I did not want to be here anymore and to start searching for some answers to some question that I was afraid to ask and worse yet afraid to hear the answers to. How does one find that thing that they can ground themselves to so they want to change? Then the issue comes when we know we have outgrown that thing that has grounded us, even though the thing has brought us back to reality. Guess it is kind of like the 12 steps . . . How many steps does it take to get someone to where they are content to not try anymore to fix things? I can't answer this because I have not found out or made it there yet. Don't think I ever will. Better to keep focused on how things are and remember how they were so that snake doesn't get me.

Yes I need to remember as much as I can so I won't try and run away. Not only in the sense of really running but also in the sense of avoiding my mind, my past, my thoughts. After all if you run away from your thought, fears, or even dealing with situations in front of you, how can you ever tackle them? Things never go away without any help. A big gust of wind might stir up some leaves if the season is right, and cover that brown patch of your lawn. That patch that always held your eyes focused to. Now it all looks the same, but is it the same or is it just a pretty dress on the wicked old wolf that if given the right opportunity will gobble you up. That wolf will always be there. That wolf will never go away. Just remembering this is a big step in the right direction. You can't forget about what is lying in wait. Keep the gun loaded. In other words keep your mind focused on the positive, enough that you can overcome any negative thought or situations that will come your way. Either that or fall prey again.

GETTING READY TO GOING HOME

FINALLY THE EVENT THAT I never thought would get here. Actually I never thought of it until the end. Easier to stay focused and do your job. You can say that the life I left behind in the states I left out of my mind. Better that way I think . . . Priorities are changing not only for me but also for all the other soldiers who are finally getting to go home to their families and their lives. The freezers and refrigerators that were once a great comity seem silly, though most of the soldiers get a quick buck from the relieving unit. Me I remember what it was like when we arrived. How there was no shower, what little water we had was far warmer then piss warm. Even the freezers when we finally got them, never really gave you the chance to drink lots of cold water. Seems the 120 to 140 degrees seem to not take much time to melt the ice and warm the water up.

For me I wish no gain from the items that I had acquired throughout the year. Even my swimming pool that my mother sent me was just given away to the new solider with a smile and a wish of good fortune. Afraid that I would change my mind and they would lose their booty he tried to force money on me. Seemed everyone else was selling theirs. Funny couldn't anyone else remember the hardship that we all endured when we first arrived on this wonderful FOB (forward operating base). No bathrooms. No showers, no water, hell no living quarters. It was a scramble to find your area to build something where you could just lay your head down. With a warm wish I laughed and said enjoy. Keep your money I am going home.

I did tell my mom that I left the pool there and just gave it away. You would think maybe she would be a little mad that I did not appreciate the gift. This was not the case. I think the fact that the pool would be there and enjoyed by other soldiers seem to please her. As such it should. I know you could tell that he really was surprised and excited about what I had left him. It would seem so little to have back at home yet a quite a lot to have over here in Iraq. Most were happy to get a refrigerator, and here I gave him a pool with a deck and a connex (metal box living quarters) fully furnished. To include protective sand bags full of scorpions all around it.

LAST MAN OUT

SOME ONE HAD TO BE the last man out of FOB (forward operating base) Orion. So I volunteered . . . something they tell you never to do. Together with Smutley (a nickname I had for a sergeant who use to be in my tow platoon years ago) we were expose to check our BN area for anything left behind and communicate with the new unit on any last minute questions that they might have. It was expose to take a couple weeks but only ended up taking four days. We then hitched a ride with a patrol going to FOB Anaconda. Our last patrol in country seemed short in ways and long in others, as the adrenalin was running through my veins. Worse than I ever thought it was before. Could I actually forget about Iraq and just enjoy a quiet ride without all the bombs and bullets flying around. No and it seemed the closer we were to getting to the front gate the more my mind was visioning the noise and smoke of the attack that was surely to come. It was uneventful as far as any action from ant coalition forces goes on the road but inside my mind it was the most dangerous ride that I was ever on.

When we finally got inside Anaconda I did relax some. Now all I had to worry about was the daily indirect fire attacks, which for the most part had no real pattern of control, mostly just rounds blindly being shot into the FOB. Still it seemed a lot more peaceful and I could almost enjoy the fact that all I had to worry about was Smutly and I catching a ride to Kuwait. Just the two of us with no real urgency to be anywhere on time . . . It was really nice and relaxing while it lasted. We did finally catch up with the last of our unit in FOB Anaconda staying in big tents with nice comfortable cots where you waited for a seat on a plane to go to Kuwait.

The wait lasted a few days and consisted of attending a couple formations a day and then just laying around trying to deal with the anticipation of finally getting on a plane and out of this country. The sirens of the indirect attacks happening on the FOB seemed to have little effect on us, and no one in our unit even runs to the barriers that have been placed around for protection from them. Laughingly we watch as others run to the safety of them. We just dumb grunts who don't want to play no more and all we can focus on is getting out of this god forsaken country.

Finally we get a chalk (military version of a boarding pass) to Kuwait on a C130. The take off was so steep you would think that they were trying to go to outer space. This steep climb is a tactic that the Air force uses to get the planes out of small arms / RPG / anti-aircraft range in a hurry. The tactic makes for an interesting takeoff. I guess getting shot at would be interesting also, maybe even a little more memorable. Though I am sure I have had enough of that already.

KUWAIT TO DRUM

KUWAIT IS JUST A QUICK stop. It's December 31ˢᵗ and the army wants us out of country before the New Year. Don't want to pay the combat pay. Great, I would gladly give it all back if I did not have to come in the first place. Something's or some places are just not worth any amount of money. So things should move a little faster now. Just fast enough to get our cards swiped logging us out of country, and then things seem to slow down. No longer is there such an urgency to get us moving. Of course as we swiped our cards we walked into a plane. Now we cannot leave the plane because we are not in country anymore. Funny if we are not in country where are we? It is like we are in Purgatory; we sit around waiting to be judged worthy of leaving, or maybe just waiting for our turn to go to the gate. So we all end up yelling happy New Year sitting on the runway locked in the plane. What a way to start the New Year.

Of course being the last plane out for the BN leaves us with a smaller number. Great not so crowded or so one would think. With every positive there always is a negative. Our negative is that with a smaller number means a smaller plane and the plane can't fly all the way to Ft Drum without refueling. First time in my life I get to yell happy New Year three times in three different countries and three different time zones. So if are standing on the Hoover Dam and think that it's great to yell happy New Year and then take a step to wait for another hour to yell happy New Year for the second time and think that it is great and is the most times that anyone can yell happy New Year you are mistaken. Wonder what the most times someone got to yell happy New Year in a single day? Maybe the astronauts get to yell it in all the times zones. Funny all the time zones at almost the same time. Instead of waiting an hour they could wait only a second. Guess that makes me look small. Of course if you out there everything looks small. Wonder if Ripley ever thought of that. It was nice to actually speak to my family from Ireland at the stroke of midnight. I mean most Irish people dream of something like this, some moment to last a life time. If only I was Irish. Well I do remember it and sure I will for a life time. Thanks Uncle Sam.

Finally we do arrive in Fort Drum, or should I say Wheeler-Sack Army Airfield. Quick gauntlets walk through all the high ranking officers and politicians, as well as a few family members. No time to waste. Outside we have a formation to account for everyone and then on the busses to Old Post on Fort Drum. Old post is just what it sounds like. It is the older wooden buildings that have been vacated by the active military and are still being used by the National Guards. Most of the buildings are in such disrepair that sometimes they condemn them for a short period of time. Like say there is too much ice on them and they are afraid of the building collapsing. Who makes these calls I do not know but I am certain that they are in a nicer brick building. They are better than a tent though.

It seems like forever, so close yet so far away. FREEDOM! Maybe have a cold beer with your Army family, or if you really lucky maybe you live close enough so that you can meet your civilian family. Of course we still don't know the schedule for out processing. Still have our weapons. Could be another you can't go anywhere by our BN commander. (Something he did a lot of before we went off to Iraq.) Only he knows why. Maybe someone out there can understand how someone would refuse soldiers on the verge of the unknown from spending what might be the last moments with their loved ones. Not this time. Secure your gear, and turn in your weapons. See you all in the morning. What? No restrictions. After all what could any of us do being so long away from our families, good fast food, opposite sex, and of course alcohol. Who am I to complain? Here you go see you later . . .

OUTPROCESSING

To my surprise processing from active duty back to National Guard did not take but a couple days. Everyone was on their own time frame. I am sure the rear detachment kept a list of who was still on active duty and who was done out processing, other than that you are on your own time schedule. When you got all the stations done you were out. You had to speak to people about what you saw and how you feel and if you have a job still waiting for you when you returned. They wanted to know what was different in your civilian life since you left. What your plans were and if you felt stable. Funny how can one know if they are stable enough to be in our society till they actually get there and see how they interacted with society? Is it also not true that you are the last one to know if you have an issue? Well I felt fine, was a state worker going to the same job, was married, and was not my first conflict. Surely I would have no problems dealing with things.

The medical screening mad me a little upset. I requested a complete physical but all I got was a piece of paper with instructions on how to file a claim and request a physical after I was home through the VA. I guess the amount of soldiers and the amount of time and space had a lot to do with this. Still I knew if I did not do it then I would not do it. Bet that was the case in a lot of us.

Seems we are all cattle and are being sent to the slaughter house. No one wants to get too close to you, just a number and keep it going. How many will suffer because they are not prepared. I should be ok. I feel like me, I am me. Nothing has changed in me. Is there some magical wand or way to regain what we had before we were deployed? Do we even care or want the same as we did before. After all how can one think that a year of indirect and direct fire everyday, bombs, pipelines being blown up, mangled bodies, the smell and even the temperatures reaching up in the high 140:s, (Yes 140 believe it or not) would affect or change someone? Its can you realize that you are different. Do you know how you are different and the big question do you believe you need help? What has to happen before you finally realize that you can't walk this path alone? I am sure everyone's story varies some but I also believe that they all follow the same type of path. When do you finally step out of your sanctuary and stand up and yell HELP.

I know it took me awhile to get to that point. It did not happen over night. Recovery or should I say some signs of some type of recovery, for is one ever really recovered, did not seem to take that long. But then again by the time I got to this point I had no idea what time was, what I did yesterday or even a desire for tomorrow. What a sad sack I was. I knew it was up or out. Sometimes I still wonder if I took the easy road or the right road. Wish I could say I don't ponder this thought anymore. But like a drug addict you always got to be on your guard, and know the signs to your triggers and what to do to reduce them. Even though sometimes that snake seems to strike without warning and leaves you little time to react.

Anyway in the Army's wisdom you go from full combat to discharge to the streets in a matter of days. Though you are eager and glad to be free from the rules and regulations, you don't think that maybe its too fast. Maybe it's too much of a jolt. I mean a couple weeks for leave are one thing. You know you are going back and you stay focused. Knowing you are done you kind of shake it off or try to shake off all of the feelings and fears that you have kept bottled up. Now you need to get them out without breaking the glass.

Maybe there should be some kind of out processing where you train on being in society? Does that sound funny? I mean the Army spends lots of money to train to get you ready for war. You would think that some more effort would be given to those soldiers going home. I mean all the classes and time spent on getting us ready to handle anything over there yet they don't take any time or effort into making sure we are prepared for life here after being there. How many families have broken up because they did not understand that their love ones have changed? Not only has the soldier in the field changed, but also help the soldier understood that their loved ones are not the same also. Some have leaned on others in more ways than one. Some have gained the confidence to do things for themselves, and some just have moved on but don't know how to tell their soldier that.

Why can't the government keep soldiers in out processing longer and make them go to classes about fitting in and how to look for triggers? Why can't significant others be brought in with their service member and go through some kind of class that even if it can't be too specific at least can give some warnings signs and some information about what is out there to help them? I am sure that it would cost a lot but it might save money in the long run, better yet it has the potential of saving lives. How much money is a life worth to the government anyway?

I did speak with my VA therapist about why so little time is spent on out processing compared to in processing. A question she said that has been discussed in some of her meetings with superiors. Who knows maybe someday there might be? If I was a betting man I would bet against it though. Easy to justify money for combat but it is a lot harder to get a budget for out processing. Maybe because all the Army trains for is war not peace. Maybe the answer lies in the VA being more involved in out processing units. Maybe the answer is having the VA come to the soldier rather than wait for the soldier to go to them. Some soldiers don't make it to the point to seek help.

MONEY PROBLEMS

Money:
- Something generally accepted as a medium of exchange, a measure of values, or a means of payment.
- Officially coined or stamped metal currency.
- Money of account.
- Coin or paper money.
- The first, second, and third place winners in a horse or dog race.
- Prize money.
- Persons or interest possessing or controlling great wealth: according to one's preference or opinion.

THE THING THAT HAS THE ability to make one happy or sad (or so most think), that money causes one to choose between right and wrong at times. Most people might think or say that the more they have the least amount of issues they will have. If only this was true. Of course there are places and times where money surely helps. Don't get me wrong I am not trying to say that money is over rated, but saying more that although money does determine a lot it should not be the sole thing that makes one tick. I mean if this is so then you would live to make money, and you would not want to spend it but make more. Is that a life? Yes it is a life to some, but it is not the life for me. Maybe because I never was in a place where there was so much that I could think like that. I think growing up to where I was not spoiled has instilled in me a quality where money is important but only to where you have the basic necessities. Of course then one would ponder what the necessary necessities are. After all now a days you got to have an IPOD, Tablet, Smart phone . . . the list goes on and on. When I grew up I had three channels on the black and white television, and a Nintendo where you could play ping pong or shoot a tank.

Being deployed the Army handles all your basic needs for you. Even if the soldiers complain that the food sucks, and it does a lot of the time, for the most part it is there. They give you a place to sleep, clothes as well as other things to put on your back. But who takes care of the family you leave behind? How can we make sure they are not going without? I can't say that the service does not try to help you on this area. They do. They give you lots of advice and have support systems set up where most issues can be handled before they get out of control. Of course the issue here is when someone knows that something is out of control and when does one get to the point that they ask for help, or do they just wait till it is too late.

Being a senior NCO (non-commission officer), making sure that my family had enough to get by did not seem to be a issue. First I took my wife's name off of my savings account, which had my direct deposit from the Army going to. I took out two allotments for both our vehicles. $1000.00 of bills she would not have to worry about. I also sent her a allotment of $1000.00 dollars twice a month. Surely someone could live on that much money with little problems. I mean in reality its $3000.00 of actual spending money a month. What does someone have to make to have that much spending money after taxes, $70,000.00 maybe? We can say a little less just to be fair to her.

Oh I forgot to say that my wife is an LPN (licensed practicing nurse) for the state of New York. She makes an easy $38,000 a year. You would think that she would have enough for whatever came her way. The question is whether there was enough money for whatever came my way?

Finding that she had enough money where she did not have to worry. Surely there should not be any bad in that? There are always unforeseen issues. The issue that she had to deal with the most though was simple in her eyes. She just plain old did not have enough time to spend the money. Yes that is what I said. How many of you would like to be in her shoes? Of course there is always the after effect. You know what goes up must come down, the saying that if this happens then that will happen. Well it plays here also. Her decision was to go part time. Works less spend more, and could she spend. Even this could have been ok if she only did one thing before she spent the money. Can you guess what it is? Believe it or not it is such a simple thing as paying bills. After all they don't go away. In reality they don't go away, in her mind I think they just never existed. Too bad that could not be reality. Or was it to her, was it her reality? Who or when will she realize that she needs to wake up or does someone have to slap her across the face for her to see the light.

Now the Army or the government tries to help its soldiers with laws and programs so military personnel and their families can have some protection while they are deployed away. Not a bad thing. But then again an indoor toilet is not a bad thing, unless of course it over flows . . . One was all bills could not be over 6% interest. Great all my credit card rates have to go down. Also with everyone being behind Enduring Freedom, most did not ask for any money due till the service person comes off active duty. Great 6% interest and they don't want any money. Of course a smart person would have made some payments if they could. Not my wife. The less they wanted the more she had . . . It was like she had Christmas all over again.

Believe it or not she went to Niagara Falls on the Canadian side with her mother and our three girls. Sounds like a good trip, what could be wrong with that? Here comes the problem though. It is raining. What do you do? Some would say that is not a problem, we go see the falls anyway, after all you do get a little wet just from the mist. Not my wife she got a better plan. How that song does goes . . . rain drops are falling on my head, and they won't defeat me I going to stay right here and out last you . . . Oh I don't think that is the way the song went, but that is how she went. She stayed in a hotel seven days till it stopped raining. Now if it was really raining and you came from long way off I might say ok. But when you live across the border only four hours away I think it is a little much. Well I can't say too much because I never saw the bill. Just the mention of it would make a grown man cry or laugh. I was no exception, although it was a laugh or cry for pity, for composure, for saneness, surely someone is not that stupid.

I did make it home for two weeks leave. Even got to go trick or treating with my kids. Halloween is my favorite holiday. I have up to this time never missed a night of trick or treating with them. I even dress up in a gorilla suits with a Cyclops mask and knock on doors myself. I do get a lot of compliments and scare a lot of small kids, Of course I play the part to the max, with crouching and limping and growling. Sometime I would even try to take the entire bowl of candy, and sometimes I would try to take the person holding the bowl of candy. The suit had two half coconuts that cover my pecks or you

21

know someone else's breast. I have gotten lots of comments on these also. I even wore slippers that had fuzzy bears on them. These were great times that I will always cherish in my mind.

While I was home I found out that my wife took $1000.00 from my savings account and had it transferred into our joint checking account. Seems the bank never turned her card off. She could not get money out but she could transfer. How or why she ever got to the point of trying this is a mystery to me. I mean it is not like I won't find out sooner or later, I mean later. I told her that I went to the bank and I fixed it so she could not do this anymore. I think she knew I never had the time, or that I did not go and do this. I should have at least called. Not too smart of me. You would also think after the way I acted when I found out she took the $1,000.00 she would not have the nerve to try this again, or at least wait a good amount of time to give her a excuse for doing this. Not her, the very day I fly off she takes $5,000.00 dollars out. Guess she showed me. Although I have to say that this was the beginning of the end of us. I had plans on taking her and me on a cruise to the Caribbean when I got back. When I found out about the last $5,000.00 dollars it sort of put an end to that.

Now I do go to the bank. Took awhile for what I was saying to register into the mind of the bank officer. Here is where I now think I should have made a different choice. Here is where I think I should have called in quits, and not tried to work on our relationship anymore. It seems now like the way I should have gone. Instead I have to bluntly say that I am still with my wife and that we are trying to make things work could you please just make it so she cannot access any more of my money. She has never had access to my money from that day on. Maybe I am getting smarter. Not smart enough yet though. I still got things to learn.

So let's sum things up

1. Both vehicles payments made. $1,000.00 a month.
2. Allotments to her twice a month $2,000.00 a month.
3. She goes part time
4. Takes $6,000.00 out of my savings.
5. Does not make payments on any bill that does not ask for any.
6. Has nothing to show for all the money that is gone.

Do you think that is bad enough? Believe it or not there is more! She gets a credit card at 5% interest for $5,000.00 in October. In February when they want 700 as a minimum payment and the rate is at 33.333% I call there in an attempt to reason with them on the rate, I find out when she got the card and that it is maxed out and better yet that she has not made a payment. I am informed that she has not had the card long enough for them to assist me with any of their programs. Can one even imagine what the interest on $5,000.00 at 33.333% rate would be in a year? WHAT THE FUCK MAN! How can this be legal? Guess some big shots gave money to the right politician. How can anyone really pay this?

Can you even imagine how mad I was when I learned all this? Now I could pay my bills and let her deal with her own knowing full well that she won't pay anything. So I decide to try and do the right thing and set out to pay off her bills first and then to get to mine.

There were so many issues dealing with her and money. It is lucky for us that I work for the state at a criminally insane hospital. A place where there is always some overtime available. So I dive into my job. Most days I am working 16 hours. Then I would drive a hour home get a little something to eat watch a little TV, try to sleep a couple hours and then drive the hour back to work to do it all again. If you can only imagine how tiring and exhausting both physically and mentally this was. Still I can't make my minimum payments. What do you do? SELL . . . SELL . . . SELL anything and everything, borrow from my retirement and sign up for programs with a credit counseling place. All this is destroying what little credit rating I had left. Of course she has a great credit rating since I cosigned on all her loans and am paying her bills off first. It takes me two years to finally catch up enough so I could take a breather. Now I can relax!

GOOD TIMES AT WORK

SOME PEOPLE THINK THAT WORK is a stressful place. The fact that I work at a mental hospital for the criminally insane should sound stressful, I guess if you think about it is really is. My opinion seemed different now then it was before I went to Iraq. I mean after all how this place could even compare to the daily stress of being over there. Here we ducked a punch here and a punch there; get called names and maybe even complaints from patients put in on us, where we might even be separated from them while the complaint is being investigated. Over there you duck indirect fire every day, IED are very normal. We could go on and talk about just the place, the weather, the bugs, the spiders, all of which I feel are a lot more stressful then working at this hospital.

Maybe that was one on the issues that I had. This place seemed different to me. It seemed to be calmer. With the money situation and the tenseness of being home and the working all the time it is no wonder that work became my happy place. It became my happy place where I can relax more than anywhere else. Does that sound funny that this insane asylum is the best place I have to relax and unwind?

I won't say that everything I did was perfect. Nor will I say that I never did anything that had to be addressed by a superior. I can say that my immediate supervisor as well as my shift supervisor adored me. Adored, maybe that's not the right word. They appreciated every time I was there. They counted on me and respected me enough to trust me with situations and the ability to make decisions. Even got a great yearly review where my shift supervisor wrote that I was her go to guy on the shift. If she had a problem she knew she could count on me to handle it without question. It felt good to be treated this way. What little issue or quarks that someone might say I had was nothing more than anyone else had and I was holding everything together.

Civil Service held a test for the next level of my series while I was in Iraq, so that when I got home I called them and inquired about me being able to take the test and be put on the list. It took a couple weeks to finally get the answer. The question had to go up the chain. I would like to think only because it took someone higher to have the authority to make this decision. None then less I can't say anything bad about the state civil service services because they did do the extra to accommodate me in taking this test and being put on the list.

When my shift supervisor heard that I was going to take the test she seemed excited and told me to "make sure you score at least a 90". I took to studding and since I was the only one taking the test there was lots of extra copies in the education and training wing. I read the book over and over again. I even had people read me the questions so we could see how I would answer them. I wanted to do a good job that I read the book over and over again. When the day came to take the test I was not nervous. Maybe I should have been. I seemed quite at ease and when I opened the book I seem to relax even more if I could of. The test seemed like a breeze. I mean most of the questions were on everyday stuff concerning your job, and some on writing skills, which was not my strong point but from all the paperwork that I did in Iraq sure seemed easy enough. When the results finally came in the mail it was a enlightening feeling when I saw that I got a 90 on it as my supervisor told me to. I can still remember the high feeling I felt. Pride just a gleaming through.

Things are looking up. I feel as though I fit in and I matter. I can and will make a difference. I feel as if I am ready maybe even longing or needing the challenge.

REALIZATION OF MY MENTAL STATE

Realization:

- The action of realizing.
- The state of being realized.
- Something realized.

Realize:

- Bring into concrete existence: accomplish.
- To cause to seem real; make appear real.
- To convert into actual money.
- To bring or get by sale, investment, or effort; gain.
- To conceive vividly as real; be fully aware of.

FINALLY I CAUGHT UP ON my bills so no more working doubles every day. What a relief. Finally I can relax and let my mind wander as it may. Of course the only problem here was that when I finally took a breather I finally start to see that I was having some shall we say difficulties? I guess you never really know what is going on if you don't stop and think about things. Who knew that sometimes thinking is not so good, or maybe the truth is that I should have thought more before. Hind sight is always so good. Trying to hold on to ones family some people would do just about anything. Unfortunately for me trying to hold on to what was there or what I remember was there maybe cost me more than if I would have just started the wheels moving us apart when I first returned from Iraq, like everyone in my family said I should have done.

So now I realize that I am not sleeping and that I am full of anger. I am full of so much anger that I even get mad at myself. Driving a vehicle is just about the worse thing you could think of to do. It is a big difference because over there you are driving someone off the road or shooting out the engine to get them out of the road. Now I actually have to try and follow the flow of traffic. Oh how easy it would be to just sideswipe them out of the way. Following a big vehicle that you can't see around just is not going to happen! The feeling is so real, and trying to unwind when you get away from them is not that easy. The "high" that your body feels puts you in a different sphere, looking out. Kind of like you are playing a video game, only the vehicles or the bodies don't mend that fast.

Now I seem to be getting more agitated with every passing day. I try to keep to myself as much as possible. I am physically kicking chairs out of my way at work. I always try to sit alone in the lineup room before work. I start to be aware that I am only getting two to three hours of restless sleep a night, but is that really sleep? Maybe it could better be described as a time out for me. When my body does finally crash and falls into a deeper sleep the nightmares come. So vivid sometimes that I bolt upright with sweat all over my face, and worse yet I come to realize where I am after hearing my wife scream or cry in pain. I was actually a little afraid to go to sleep, which surely gave me less sleep, and made me more irritable to everyone including even to myself.

Where does one turn? Would it not be easier to just say fuck it and do the deed that my mind ponders more and more often every day? Just take my Remington 629 44 magnum revolver and BANG! How much would it really hurt? Would I feel it at all? Would I even hear the shot? Would anyone really care? Would anyone really miss me?

Close it came. How close I guess depends on your opinion. To me it got to one step away. I actually have held the loaded pistol a couple times to my head. Even though I wanted to die, wanted the pain and the loneliness to go away, I always did seem to find one thing to live for. One more thing that will help gives me the strength to help me make it through to another day. Maybe I can just make it through one more day of hell. There is a funny thing about another day because I have lost track of time. Could not remember yesterday and what I did. I had no desire about what tomorrow would bring. I could not think of anything that I wanted to accomplish in the future. What a sad sack I had become.

Somewhere in this time frame is when I started being nice to my co-worker. It kept my mind off of me and onto something else, someone else. Finally realizing that things needed to change and with me having no desires of my own, her desires became mine. She became my life. She seemed to be motivated by me giving her so much attention. She wanted me to be her ken doll. Wanted to mold me to be her BFF, or maybe just wanted me to be everything that she was missing out of her life, she wanted to feel she was the most important thing in the world to me. I blindly followed. I gave up my soul, my existence, all I was is a piece of clay that needed to be molded and now I had a person to mold me. Mold me into something better than what I was. It turned out to be the beginning of the end of one chapter and the start of another. At least now I have a let off valve. I have a focuses on something besides me and my misery. Maybe this is why I fell so hard and became so blinded to everything and everyone except her.

Does this sound terrible? I mean what about my kids? How could a parent not think about them? Deep down they were always there in my mind. Like a lighthouse in the distance on a foggy stormy night. They were there to guide me every now and then but for the most part did not seem to care. Her life became my life. It was a new beginning and a new end. It gave me a better tomorrow and some thoughts of something to look forward to if only for later today, it was a start. Who knows maybe I might remember something about yesterday tomorrow?

Got a friend and I started to pick up on her habits. One of her bad habits was of drinking. Drinking which started me on a different road with different problems. Even though it felt so right, so much like it was solving my problems with fitting in, it was just pushing them further and farther away with every bottle. It was pushing them further away with my new problems in front of them. Would I ever see this? Could I ever come to realize what I was doing before I did something I could not take back? Did I even care? No. All I cared about was my time with her, and my time drinking with her.

REACTION AFTER REALIZATION

Reaction:

- A response to a stimulus or the condition resulting from such a response
- A contrary or opposing action.
- A political tendency to oppose progress or favor a return to former conditions.
- A chemical transformation or change.
- Physics—A nuclear reaction.

LIKE THE SAYING GOES FOR every action there is a reaction. Every decision has pros and cons, and the same goes for trying to get a handle on you. If you think you don't matter just try and clear your mind and watch someone in your life that you love and maybe you can see maybe you can realize that it is not just you that is hurting, and when / if you get to the point where you are ready to change to try and fix you. You will also have to be ready to deal with others. To help others deal with you especially if these people are in your immediate family / circle.

The fixing of my marriage was easy in ways and tough in others. I did try and save it one, two, maybe even three times too many. I was afraid how my kids would react. Now I think that maybe I made things worse by trying to make it work.

When I left for Iraq my girls were 7, 9, and 11 years old, which is still very young. I left when my girls would still run out shouting "DADDY, DADDY'S HOME" whenever I got there. It is one of the things that I think of the most. Funny something so simple and easy and yet the glow they had and the passion that I felt still lingers on in my mind.

I was out of their everyday lives for half of 2003 and all of 2004, but when you take into account working mostly doubles for the next two and a half years you could maybe see where the miscommunication or lack of communication lies. Worse was still to come because when I started doing the running around and the drugs I took away what little time I could have spent with them away. When I finally came to see what I had become and started the long climb back to reality I had to put myself first. Not to say that I did not attempt to rebuild my relationship with my daughters and even my wife. For the kids it was a slow moving train, and for my wife it was a fast rolling steam roller. Not fast enough for me. Although I did try one last time and I did give her 100% of my effort. Lucky for me we both knew that there never would be any trust either way.

ATTACHING TO SOMEONE

Attach:

- To fasten or become fastened; connect.
- To bind by ties of affection or loyalty.
- To affix or append: attached her signature to the contract.
- To seize by legal writ.

EVERYONE SOONER OR LATER ATTACHES to someone or something or they cease to be of this world. Being of this world sometimes does have its appeal at times. I surely needed something or someone to attach myself to. Someone or something to make my mind work or think of something besides of bills, working all the time, or dealing with the wife, or shall we say the stress of her and I being near one another, which has only grown more and more with the time passing and our inability to effectively communicate to an agreement of our money issues not to mention the fact that I don't believe either of us would be able to commit to following anyway.

The more time that I was spending at work, the more it was beginning to feel like it was my safe place. It was the safest place for me in my mind. How funny is that, a maximum secure mental health hospital for the criminally insane is my safe place in the world? What is wrong with me? Maybe I belong in a place like this! I am sure you could get a few to agree with that statement.

Everyone has their own story and their own issues and concerns. Sometimes they clash with others; because of this my ward swapped an SHTA (security hospital treatment assistant) with another one. To me it did not really matter. The one that was leaving us in my mind was a lazy sloppy worker maybe because they were older or maybe because they just did not care either way. If it was a team sport and I was choosing the teams I would not pick either of them. The SHTA that we were getting was as far as her reputation goes a trouble maker. It would be a tossup between the two. The winning factor was that the one being assigned to my ward was far more enjoyable to look at. I could even go as far as to say that she was downright desirable to me

So when she did show up you could see the discontent in her voice and see it in her posture towards everyone including the patients. When she lashed out at me I right from the start did what I told my SRSHTA (senior security hospital treatment assistant) I was going to do and gave it right back to her. I did not give her any breaks. Maybe because of her maybe more because of me and what I was going through in trying to deal with my life at this time.

This went on for some time. A few months I think, don't really know what was different on the day that things changed. I do recall that for a brief moment I did not think of my troubles. My mind was freed just long enough to see what was going on. What I saw was this very miserable hot sexy woman who was being rudely talked to and treated by everyone. Once I saw this I kept a mental note to watch and observe her more. LOL . . . More, I sure did not mind watching her more! My conclusion was that if anyone was treated as she was being treated by all anyone would have a hard time acting any other way then she was. How could one be nice while taking so much hospitably from every direction? I would not be mean to her anymore. I was going to go out of my way to be nice to her from now on.

I made the first step toward stopping the tension between her and me by simply being nice and saying nice things to her. The first time she looked as if she was going to fall over and cry, but then lashed out again at me. I did not waver. I told myself that no matter what she did I would be nice to her. I would be her candle in the night. I would be her shining light in another wise gloomy night. Ruder and ruder she got those next couple days to me. I kept a smile and a nice if not sexual comment back to her. I could notice her attitude toward me lesson as time went on and I remained nice to her and then it started to change to where I would even get a friendly comment now and then from her. Soon we even began speaking to one another just because we could and not because we had to. Then we started working together as a team. We made each other's day better and easier.

It progressed to the point where we would talk about going out after work for a drink or two. Something that I knew I would love to do but it also was something that I was afraid to do. I was afraid to enjoy life. One day we were leaving at the end of our 3-11 shift and we ended up walking out together. Flirting all the way to her vehicle and even asking and receiving a chance to hop in and go out with her. So close it was but at the last second instead of stepping in her Honda CRV I instead said goodbye and went to my car, with some stupid cop out line.

All the way on my way home and still through the night all I could think of was what if? What if I did get in the car? What if the night would progress our relationship? The excitement and desire was running through me. I was feeling things that I forgot existed, and I told myself never again would I say no to any invitation from her for any togetherness we might share, no matter how harmless, and all I could see was her and I wrapped in each other's arms in physical bliss. Even if it was farfetched or so I thought.

My opportunity came a few short or long days later. Short in time but forever in my mind. She was sitting in the doorway to the dayroom reading a book "Diaries of a Black Woman" I believe. I asked her what she was reading and she showed me. With a joking but hopeful remark I asked her to tell me all about her fantasy or her idea of the perfect night. I told her that she could think on it and email me it later. My mind whirled when she said she would. The excitement was boiling inside of me! Longing to read what she would write and how I could maybe use it to my benefit. Hopefully she was not joking or playing with me. Surely she would not let her guard down so openly to me.

The next day there it was on my work email. I was scared yet curious to see what she possible had written to me. Yes the desire and anticipation was so deep that it consumed me and every day I could not think straight and I longed for it more and more. The high was short lived and the disappointment set in hard when I read what she had sent to me. What she had promised me was exactly what she desired and wanted, but what I got was a blanket memo form statement about how a guy needs to last longer then so many minutes and how she hates this and that. It could have been a PG statement in a book about sex for 5th graders. It had no real details and was not personalized in any way. My excitement turned to disappointment which caused my frustration and anger to arise inside of me. I made the move to have a chance to change our relationship status into something more and I felt like I was being taunted even laughed at. What a rude way to be turned down. Almost enough to give up, but I was so focused in my mind about trying any and everything possible to achieve the goal that I set my sights on and that I would stop joking around about it like a school kid and tell her what I really felt and what was on my mind.

So vivid and detailed was my response to her that when she wrote back all she could say was "WOW I NEVER KNEW!" I let her know how I could not get her off my mind and how I desired her so. I spoke of how I regretted not getting in her car and how I wondered what would have happened if I did get in the car that night. How I would do any and everything that she desired no matter what the cost was. I gave examples of what I would do, how I would do it. I left nothing out for any imagination to think on. I put all my feelings of desire and longing to forgo any more childish foreplay and to go right to the prize. No cost was too high for me to pay or bear to help me get there.

It sort of took all of the wondering for her with me expressing myself in such details. It sort of took all the wondering for her about what I was thinking. It would still be a couple weeks more before our schedule allowed for us to consummate our relationship. This did not stop us from growing closer and asking specific information about one another. My desire was growing every time we spoke. Finally it was the first time in the last four years I could remember me anticipating doing something. Was she being truthful with me, or was she just leading me on? Even though I did think of this I was done being soft spoken about what I was thinking of.

I even offer to go to a hotel with her and that I would pay for it. I thought maybe it would be easier since she was also married, but she flatly turned me down on this. Maybe she wanted to stay in a comfort zone for her in the beginning. I don't know, but it was not long before she would be alone at home. Or should I say would have been alone if I did not show up.

Show up! Funny it was not really like that. Seems she was worried about her neighbors telling her husband some strange vehicle was in the driveway. Seemed like she did not want me to know where she lived. So I parked miles from the house in a hospital parking lot and rode with her. Stranger yet was the fact that she made me hide in the back of her car with my head down until she was inside her garage and the lights to the door opener finally turned off. Awkward to say the least but it did also make it seem that much more exciting to me.

34

So we get inside and she wants to shower and change her clothes. She also makes me shower. Not a bad idea because we just came from work. Then she wants to go out and get something to eat and drink. Are her nerves working with her, MAYBE? I WAS DONE WAITING AND I SPOKE MY MIND, Instead of food drink, and then sex, I want sex, food, drink and more sex. She just laughed at me and said to relax, but I was like a tiger or so I acted and I was posed to strike. Strike I did, wanting to make sure she was happy with my performance I dove right in and ate away till she could stand it no more. Then she asked for me to be in her and I could not say no. IT WAS A DREAM. This could not be true. Yes it was and forgets the dream this was heaven. So engrossed was I in making a lasting impression (in the hopes of repeat performances) that when she became the aggressor underneath me I stopped in mid stroke in disbelief. For a moment I was lost and the moment seemed like a eternity. What do I do? What the hell is going on? How I wanted to fuck her good and now she was the fucker and I was the one being fucked. Gathering my composure I knew I had to take control back from her. And then it was on.

The road to being whole again was starting to come into focus. Still had a long ways to go but like a pre-game speech I now was focused in the direction that the coach wanted me in. The coach had me in the direction of getting me out of a rut and claiming myself for me again, or so I thought.

14

LOSING TOUCH WITH ALL ELSE

LIFE IS FINALLY LOOKING UP, and it is about time. Maybe it was not the direction of the way it was going but more the structure of following the wants and desires of my new found friend. I don't think of this as a bad thing, even today I feel as if she was the spark that my brain needed to kick starts it. It did. She did kick start me both physically and mentally. There were a lot of times I did not agree with her wants and wishes but she always won in the end. Making her happy made me happy so I did everything I could to make her happy. Things that her husband should have been doing were now being done by me. Not just the physical part. I helped with the moving of her son's apartment, and I also was the one who was helping her with her grandbaby. Even the everyday conversations, and spending time playing cards and laughing around the outdoor fire pit.

The times that I did finally make it back to my wife and kids got less and less as the stress there grew and the relief of being with my new friend grew. My wife would ask me where her husband is. Why are you doing this? You could at least call when you are not coming home? Which only made things worse? First I would make excuses about having to help, being tired from overtimes and it was easier to just stay there. Don't want to drink and drive. Her answer to drinking and driving was I should know what I can and can not handle and stop so I could drive home. Farther and farther we were growing apart. Neither her nor I was willing to see the others side enough to try and understand where either of us was coming from. I was done. I just did not have the energy to officially put an end to my marriage.

My relationships with my kids seem to drift apart. Even my closeness to my youngest seems to drift apart. She and I use to do everything together. She would sit in my deer blind and bleat and rattle horns to lure the deer in. She always seems excited to just watch hunting shows together. A lot had to do with me being gone more and more, but it also was the fact that my wife was bad talking me to them. Telling them how I was deserting them and running around and that I did not care about them. I never once spoke badly about their mother to them, nor did I try and explain my side of the story to them. Rather I just let them make their own decision on what was what. Maybe this was not a good idea, but in my mind I was searching for something, but yet I did not want to face or recognize any of the issues that were in my life. To speak of them would be to recognize them or face them and that meant I would have to deal with them, something that I was not wanting or even able to handle at this time.

My mother did tell my youngest later on about the money and what my wife had done and was doing. She tried to explain to her my side. This was something that I was not willing to do. My mother told me that my daughter cried when she heard this. I have always tried to talk openly to my kids, at least about their lives and drugs and sex. I know I embarrassed them many times by asking them direct questions even with their friends no matter which one or which sex of them was around. My youngest did come to me and ask me about the money and what was going on. I asked her what she heard and where she heard it from. I tried to explain that I did not think it was right for a parent to bad mouth another to their kids even if the other one was doing it. I said that her mother had her own problems she was dealing with just as I did and for her not to judge her mother too harshly.

For as much as I did not want to face my issues, I wanted to be there for their issues. I wanted them to know that I did care. Sounds funny but I did care, and as much as my new friend at work has given me the spark I needed to live if it was not for my kids I would have never been around for her to help me. Yes my kids were my life raft as I was swept down that fast stinky congested sewer. The thought of them being told or finding about how I had given up was just too much for me to think about. Their smiles were always the last thing that was on my mind when I held that 44 to my head. Their smile always won. They always made me feel ashamed for what I was thinking. They always made me hate myself for what I had become, and their smiles always was what stopped me. Not enough for me to grab a hold of the steering of the raft but enough to just hold on and see where I ended up.

What I needed was to be led like a baby. I needed to be shown the ropes of life again. Shown how to walk and stand up on my own. Well stand up by leaning on someone really. This was not a bad thing in ways. The more involved in her life I became the more of life I was living, even if it was not my life it was a life. Like a dog I became part of her family. I was even soon to meet her husband and go places with them. More and more time I was spending with her and less and less was I spending in my old life.

Things steadily grew into a strong relationship with both her and her husband. Like a member of the family I was invited to go along. Each of them in their own ways gained something from me. As much as I needed them they needed me. I kept her company and happy and he was free to do whatever it was he wanted to do. He had to know that there was more going on then she said was going on between us. I did not even care, though I did ask her time and time again to tell him the truth. The more I grew to like him the more I hated what we were doing. Not enough to give it up though. I wanted what he had or what I thought he had. He had to know that there was more going on. I did not care. I asked her to tell him everything. The more I grew to like him the more I hated what we were doing. Not enough to give it up though. I wished his life was mine. I wanted what he had or what I thought he had.

So comfortable I became with them that it felt so natural. It felt so right. It felt like home. I felt secure. Secure enough to relax and enjoy the moment. The moments that I knew were not mine in reality, but in my mind it was my reality. I refused to acknowledge what my reality really was. I refused to think of that stressful place where my wife and kids were. I was lost in a new world. Lost in her world and I was totally fine with that. Or at least I was totally unconcerned about anything else but her world. She was the queen of my world. I was her jester who would jump at her command.

Even today I sometimes think that maybe I would still be caught in her world if things did not change. Just like always the change came. I knew it would come, and I could feel it inside of me. Slowly it was creeping into my world. Occasionally I would feel the difference. Yet like everything else in the real world I refused to face it. Refused to stand up on my own and shout what the fuck is this! So I stayed on my raft floating further and further down the path to total destruction. I stayed the jester. I wanted to remain the jester. Did not want to lose what I had. I had a comfort zone where I could go through life like I was living. This jester smiled to the world even as it laughs at me. Even as the world shows that I was nothing more than someone else's clown.

Maybe she thought that she had me chained down for good. Maybe she thought that I would always be there. Like the stepping stool in the corner, I was called upon and stepped upon on without thinking if I could handle the weight. Could I handle the weight of being nothing more than hers to step on? Yes I was hers, but was she mine. She would say she was, even show she was if the situation allowed it. In the beginning this was fine, but as time went on her attention turned to other things. She always focused on her issues. On her problems, and there always seemed to be another one right around the corner. She always had a excuse to keep me away from my real family. This was fine with me, up to the point where I finally realized that I was there for her but she was not there for me. Oh sure she would say that she was there, but she was not helping me overcome or even address any of my issues.

It came slow. At least in my mind it came slow. She would get mad whenever I drove home. And when I did drive home she would have a reason not to text her. She would come up with reasons why I should stay there and forget about anything else. Her affection even seemed to dwindle. Just like a marriage it seemed like it became a chore to her. The excitement and the passion became fewer and farther in time. She would give in to my pestering about some closeness, about not wanting to have sex anymore. She would give in and say "hurry up". This only made things worse. Only made me go through the motions of enjoying the sex, but the truth was that it was not the sex that I craved. It was the emotional stimuli that I wanted, needed, and longed for. Slowly at first my mind would float about being somewhere else or doing something else. Even doing nothing and becoming nothing again. Yes those thoughts started popping up more and more about me hurting myself. It seemed like more and more I was feeling like the loser again. Feeling like the fool all over again.

How can I forget about everyone and everything else and be there for her if she is not going to make me feel like I matter to her? How come my devotion cannot be returned by her? How come she makes me feel stupid for thinking of my family? How come all she wants' me to do is to be there for her? How can this help me? Why can't she see how her putting me second or third time after time again is bothering me?

The last straw came one day when I was going to my real family and I called her to talk to her. We use to talk all the time about anything and everything. The phone was always at our sides. We always kept the phone close to keep us together when we were apart. Not this time. This time she told me that she did not want to talk to me if I would not come back to her, and then she rudely hung up the phone. She refused to answer when I called her back. She ignored me as long as she could and then she did it. She turned off her phone. No longer was that tie there. I felt it snap on this day. This day stands out as the day that I knew that living for her was over and that I had to move on. To what, to where I did not know but she had taken me as far as she could and now I was being swept away again. I was being swept away to the septic pool. How long could I stay afloat? How long before I went under to never be seen again?

15

DRUGS AND ALOCHOL

WHAT A MAGICAL THING THEY can be. They can make one who feels like they don't fit in to feeling like everything is going great. Or maybe it is just an illusion that one believes to be true. Not me, I knew what they were doing to me and at the time they felt so right. They were in a way a crutch. They were something to help a cripple move around. I was the cripple and they did help me move around. They did help me start to feel like I could fit in again. Or at least fit in enough to let me keep the show going. The show that I was keeping going was my life.

I did not start out with the idea that the drugs and alcohol were the answer. It started because of who I was with. It was because of who I clung to, the person who gave me the much needed spark in my life to think that something was wonderful or could be wonderful again. Like a car with a dead battery. I needed a good jump to get me back in the game. She was there giving me that jump and a lot more.

Slow in the beginning. A drink here a drink there. With each passing day they seem to taste better going down. Easier and before I knew it some one who never really drank before was fitting in at the bar scene. I was enjoying the laughter, the throwing of darts, and just the loudness of the place. All these things seem to help. Help. Funny now I can say that the help they gave me was just plain old relief.

Relief:
- A lessening of pain or discomfort ; ease
- Something that reduces pain or discomfort
- Aid, as money, or food, given to the aged, or unfortunate
- Release from a job, post, or duty.
- Figures or forms that project from a flat background as in sculpture.
- Variations in elevation of a region.

The relief to me came from not letting my mind think for its self. Not only did it make me numb, but it also kept my mind busy so it never really had a chance to address any of the issues that were growing. Funny how can they grow if I don't recognize them? Growing like an ant hill in your back yard. If you fail to go in the back yard is it really there. Does it grow if you don't notice it growing? Maybe you could cover it up with something. If it is out of your sight then is it out of your mind. What a wonderful thing that can be. Being out of your mind . . . LOL . . . BEING OUT OF YOUR MIND!

Of course this did not change anything, nor should I say change anything for the good. Although at the time it was good. Good for me. Good for me to feel again. Yes even though in ways it numbed me or my senses it also at the same time made me feel. I felt the desire to actually want to be there. Wanted and longed for the time when I could pop a top and no one would notice anything different about me then the other people next to me.

Problem is though how do I recognize the problems, that I have or the problems that are arising now that I am numb from the drinking, do I even know that I am using it as a crutch. To me all I thought was that I was with someone who made me want to be with them. Someone I gave the power over me to. I gave the power to mold me into their perfect friend. I was a person who will be with and do anything for them till the end of time. At the time it was heaven. It was what I needed. It was the light at the end of the tunnel. The tunnel that was not the end it was the beginning. Like a baby waiting to be born. My eyes started to open like a woman's legs to let the new born life out. All I needed was a few good pushes. Hopefully the pushes will be in the right direction.

Of course negative actions only create negative results. Being around harmful things sooner or later will be harmful to you. Such was the case with the alcohol. Maybe you can say that alcohol is not harmful but if not used correctly it can be. In this case it was not regulated except by the time that it was available. So transfixed I became not only on the alcohol but also fitting in with the one who started me with the drinking. Not to say it was her fault. For even though it was negative it was also positive. Well at least in the beginning it was. More positive then anything was in my life at that time, or so I believed.

The bar scenes turned into after hour parties. If you ever been to after hour parties you know that alcohol is not all that is being done there. Of course not wanting to be the odd ball when the time came and the joint was passed around and offered, it just seemed like the right thing to do.

The quick flash of wrongness did not hold a chance of me saying no. Down lower and lower I went. Or was it higher and higher? The higher I got not only in amounts but also in occasions. What started out as a puff here and a puff there became buying a bag here and buying a bag there.

As with the alcohol the pot turned into a crutch. It was an easier crutch to use before work, during work, after work. Sometimes you just needed that edge off. The mind was tricked into relying on the numbness. Or was I the one that was tricked for it made handling things seem easier. Or so I thought. The truth was I was not handling anything any easier. It was a band aid or maybe it was some duct tape. It was the fix it all in my world. A little here a little there and everything is held inside. Of course that is what I wanted. I was too afraid to address any of them. At least not to the point that I felt I needed some help. Hell things were getting better. Better and easier.

Puff . . . Puff . . . Puff . . . DO YOU WANT SOME?????????

So now I am drinking, and smoking pot a lot. You can see how life was starting to be more fun. Or so it seemed. Laughter even if it was drug induced sure was better then dealing with reality. It was better than dealing with the road rage. Hell rolls me up another one. Driving was fun, even challenging. Have you ever gotten lost on the road you live on? Just keep driving sooner or later you will know where you are. Hopefully if you keep driving, just keep driving.

Maybe it would of gone on like this longer if things did not change. Just like the weather things always change and there was no exception here. Was it really changed or was it merely just another chapter of the same story. My story was just trying to stay numb, trying to stay numb to the world and not deal with any of the issue that I really don't want to face. I was ashamed to face. Like that old ant hill things just did not go away. They were there and they were growing. Growing in ways of how much more could be kept inside. Now some aggression was being released here and there. Maybe the aggression was not all in a positive manner but yet enough so that I kept up the show of doing my normal routine. Now instead of letting off a little steam before I blew my top I was covering up everything by staying numb. This could not last forever, unless I gave up on everything else and just enjoyed the drugs and alcohol, and the numbness that was becoming my life.

16

MAKING A CHANGE

Change:

- To make difference in some particular: transform.
- To replace with another: switch.
- A fresh set of clothes.
- Money in small denominations received in exchange for an equivalent sum in larger denominations.
- Money returned when a payment exceeds the amount due.

CHANGE, SOMETIMES IT IS FOR the better and sometimes it is for the worse. I was not to the point where I even recognized that I had a problem, or at least did not want to admit it to myself. Thought that I was doing ok, hanging in there and that things around me were shitty and I was trying to work with that rather then the truth that I was standing in sewage and that it was piling up higher and wider and was really starting to smell. People were noticing it. Others were. Still I told myself I was in control when truly I was not, and the one that I was leaning on was now dragging me deeper in my hell. It was like signing that contract with the devil himself. At first you get everything that you think you need to make you happy. Everything there is. Then you realize that the price you are paying is a big one, and yet you don't know what to do about it. So you just go along with the flow. You go along with the flow of the sewer. At least you are moving. It does not smell as bad when you are moving. It is going to be better just around the bend. The question is whether it is this bend or the next bend that it will get better. Can't get much worse right?

The change that came was just another form. Another form of something to keep you headed down that path that you don't want to cross. The form came in like a cloud. Not a cloud of smoke but a nice white round beautiful thing that could be shaped anyway you wanted. It could be used in different ways. Abused in different ways and it solved some of the problems that the drinking and the smoking created.

It was just another average night. There was nothing out of the ordinary of the smoking and the drinking. There it was. A nice shinning mirror covered with the white glowing cloud. No not a cloud of smoke but a nice row of snort of coke. OH NO! What do you do? It's not even a question of if you will or won't. Of course you know the answer here. After the first snort it was all over. I found a new friend. I found a better friend. It was a much easier friend to hide and who worked easier and faster. It was a much easier friend to hide your trouble away with. It was easier to consume and to hide. If things are not going so good just a little pinch will do you. Was it the right place right time, or was it the wrong place wrong time? Depends on how you look at it.

By this time I am feeling fine and would do anything to keep the time going. After the first snort it was all over. I found a new wonderful friend. Still the path and the stench of the sewer line continue to grow stronger. The current just keeps pulling you along. I was enjoying the ride. I was going faster and farther into my hell. So far that I start to but my own and soon I was becoming the center of attention. Or rather the focal point to where one can enjoy the richness that has become of my world. Trips down to New York City became more frequent. First to Yankee games with an extra stop to get my fix to just going for the fix. We would drive down spend the night then drive back. Nights there were not boring. Fun filled exciting times that I absorbed over and over again. I was riding the current. Who would ever want to get off the trip?

As the use of this new friend continued to grow so did the way it was enjoyed. No longer just snorting it now I am adding it to the pot and smoking it. What a different kind of high. Seem to be stronger and last longer. Was it true or was it just true in my mind. Either way it doesn't matter to me because I enjoyed it just the same. Not only did the coke find a new use but also so did the pot. We went from smoking it to eating it. Nice cookies so easy to make yet so wonderful. Hell by the time you get stoned enough off the cookies to get the munchies it was all over. Now you really enjoyed them that much more. Fill that tummy, quench that desire. By the time you ever know what is going on you are wasted beyond belief, and still your body is consuming what you just ate. Wow this high really does last. Not to mention easier to do than anything else is to do while you are driving down the road. Who would ever suspect that the wonderful cookies are such a nice treat?

So we go on. We go on stronger than before. We are able to handle much more stress in life. We are able to ignore much more stress in life. Just like that ant hill still the issues I am hiding from grow. They grow not only in size but also in numbers. Now the drugs are controlling me almost as much as that person that I am clinging to that brought me to this point. At least I was living, or was I slowly dying?

17

ISSUES AT WORK

EVERYONE IN ANYPLACE HAS SOME kind of issue sooner or later. I surely am not an exception to this rule. In the beginning I can honestly say now that I did not see some of the things that others saw about me and the way that they saw them. Surely you are always the last one to know anything about yourself. Maybe it was because I had blinders on. Maybe it was because I did not want to deal with how my life had changed since going to Iraq. Things just did not seem the same nor was my willingness or desire to come to face these changes head on.

I turned my attention away from my homestead. Away from that so called wife of mine that all I could think of was how to really hurt her, maybe in such away that I would never have to deal with her ever again. To say that I did not ponder doing her in would be a lie. I did ponder that choice as much as I ponder the choice of doing me in. The only difference was that I never did hold a gun to her head. Good thing because I know I would not have stopped.

In stead I chose to work as many hours as I could in the attempts to catch up on the bills so that maybe I could relax and take a breather. What a fool I was because no sooner did I get caught up on the bills did she charge another $25,000.00 in credit card bills that I was forced to pay half of at our divorce. Even though I wanted nothing to do with that homestead, but I also did not want to upset my kids in their lives. Another catch 22 that surely had no chance of happening but I chose to not come to terms with it yet.

Maybe I was not the model employee that I thought I was. Maybe I did have some issues that needed to be addressed. I can say that I did not have the amount of mental strength then, and was not at my peak performance, but I did attempt to change things for the better. My facility should have followed its own policy and assisted me or better yet they should have sought me out when I returned from Iraq to make sure of my mental status. Had they done this maybe things would have been better, but all they did was say welcome back and threw me to the wolves. Maybe just maybe if they would have put forth a little effort or show of concern for me I never would have held that 44.

The cold hard fact is that I had made a lot of bad decisions when I got back for all the right reasons. When I tried to crawl back to being a stable civilian all I got from the one place that should have shown me the way was closed doors, and laughs. I did take things personal, after all how was I to take them. I was not a part of the click and because I spoke my mind I was a tumor that upper management wanted to cut the life out of. It is fortunate for me that I found the strength to live to another day. I found a reason to stand on my feet and say that I would not accept being treated like this.

The more that I found closed doors at work the more it pissed me off. At first I reacted to them, but I later learned to not react too them. I now know that things there for me will never be on a honest or fair level with everyone else. I went through every agency and every department that I could think of to get someone to finally stand by my side. In the end I had to pay a lawyer to sue. The truth is though no matter what the outcome, and no matter what the amount of settlement will be, it is a tragedy for everyone. I have already lost not only my self confidence in the fairness in the leadership of upper management as well as in the AA sector. This facility as well as the state has lost my respect and my devotion. I am now just a number who cares little for their policies, and procedures. Let their poor leaders do as they must. I watch my back and long for the day when I don't have to come here anymore.

It is a crying shame that I have devoted so much time, effort, and so many years to a country and a thinking of a way of life to be cast away as if I was nothing more then a piece of shit on their boots. No wonder people act out as violently as they do. Sometimes it seems like the only way to be heard. Just like that child that acts out for some attention, so do we act out in order to be heard.

Lucky for me I found the strength through the right people and the right medication to speak out in a way that I don't have to lose my future. Though I feel that I have lost some of my integrity, I can honestly say that this facility has lost more then I have. Too bad they will never open their eyes to see the real harm that they do to others. They manage watching criminals here but they are the real criminals. They stole my sole away from me but I refuse to lie down to them. I will stand my ground to the end. For me there can be no other way, I fought for me and have found a little of a light at the end of the tunnel.

You be the judge if you dare. Just remember that things are written in my eyes and I might not know all the answers or all the reasons but if you set my story up on the wall you can only come to the decision that I was denied the opportunity, and was never given any reason. I did not do as John did, though it was close. Fuck you all in this place that destroys people's dreams as if they are nothing.

CIVIL SERVICE

LIKE I SAID BEFORE I work at a state mental hospital for the criminally insane, and it is my happy place. It was my happy place, where I felt the most comfortable and at ease. Work was holding me together. With all my money problems the fact that I could work all the over time that I wanted sure did give me some relief. Work became my life. I was just a robot going in everyday working a double to go home and do it all over again. My SRSHTA, and my shift supervisor loved me and made me feel important and wanted. My interaction with the patients was warm and friendly as much as possible. There were moments when I had to do some hands on, I guess it comes with the job, but as much as everything else in my life was a shambles at least this place was secure and I felt at ease.

My shift supervisor spoke to me about a senior item and if I was on the list. When I told her that I was in Iraq when it was taken she suggested that I get hold of civil service and see if they would let me take the test and be put on the standing list. I guess it was worth a shot. What do I have to lose? So I went to civil service and I asked about the test. The lady at the desk did not know but we filled out the papers and she was going to send them higher. It took about 3 weeks but in the end I was approved to take the test, and was given a test date. I started studying all the time. I went to the library at work and got a study guide. Over and over I read it. I had people ask me questions. Anything I could do I did to prepare myself for the test. When my supervisor learned that I was taking the test she told me I needed to get at least a 90 on it.

When the day came for the test came I seemed at ease. I tried to rest as much as possible. I was as ready as I could be and I was ready to take it. The civil service people who were given the test were very nice and helpful to me. I got all set in the room I was expose to go to and sat about half way back on the left side. Only a few other people took test there that day and none of them were taking the one that I was taking. The civil service ladies wished me good luck when I told them that I was getting the chance to take this test because I was in Iraq when it first came out. The test seemed easy. I could not believe how fast I breezed through it. I felt like I did a great job, only time would tell now.

It took a couple months before I received the letter in the mail with my score. I got a 90! Just like my supervisor said to do. I felt on top of the world, I even skipped a little. My score was placed on the list which put me in the top scores. Things are looking up, at least as far as work goes.

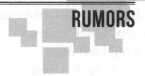

AROUND MARCH OF 2006 THE facility promoted six people to SRSHTA. All of them had the same score as I. I was a little disappointed but I did not feel any other bad feelings toward the promotions. Late in 2006 I heard rumors that people who scored less than me were being approached and asked if they were interested in being promoted to SRSHTA. I was concerned because I was not approached by anyone so I wrote my security chief to discuss my concerns.

Chief

I heard many rumors running around about openings for a grade 16. People who have scored less then I have stated that they have been asked if they are interested in a position or not. I was wondering if this means that I am going to be passed up for the job. If this is the case I would like to know the reason for me not being considered for the job. I can see nothing negative in my work performance, or am I missing something.

Thank you for your time in answering me.

Dennis,

Sorry for the delayed response as I have been away and am still trying to catch up. At this point there have been lots of rumors floating but no approval for any Sr. positions. I am however trying to add some additional items. The discussions that have taken place with folks on the list were simply to assess their interest in the position and there have been no offers made. Debbie has previously indicated that you were interested. Should additional items get approval then the offers will be made based on a consensus of Supervision. Thanks for your interest.

EARLY IN 2007 ONE MORE person was promoted to SRSHTA again they had a score of 90. Not too many 90's are left. Surely my time is coming soon. A month later they rehired one of the ones who was already promoted but gave it up and four people with a score of 85. What the fuck. What about me. A new test was given and now they are promoting people under me before the new scores take effect. So I went to our security chief and asked him why I was passed up and what I could do to better my work performance since I was confused because I always got good reviews. He told me he did not have a job for me, but gave me no other information. This was very frustrating to say the least. Not only did I not get the respect to be at least spoken to about getting or why I was not getting a job and the only answer I get is no answer. If you think I was upset over that, two days later they promoted two more people with a score of 85 to SRSHTA. Talk about insult on top of insult. I guess you can gather that with everything else going on in my life and work being my happy place and then being treated like this by upper management kind of took my breath away. It was the straw the broke the camel's back.

I could no longer hold my frustration at the world back anymore. My happy place became the very hell that I was keeping away from while at work. I tried to keep it together but I know that I must have shown my frustration. I became withdrawn at work. One of my co-workers spoke to our shift supervisor about me. She called me into her office and asked how I was doing. I told her I was trying to hold it together but it was hard. She suggested that I go to the day shift so my work performance could be seen by the day shift supervisors. I spoke to her on how I thought it was wrong for me to not get promoted and that I preferred not to go to days because it would disrupt my babysitting schedule. She gave me some extra time off to get my head on straight.

NEW BOSS

SOON AFTER THIS MY SRSHTA retired. Of course the way things were going at work it could only get worse. Now they assign a person who was newly promoted and who scored less than me over me. I tried to make the best of it even though it was killing me inside. When my new senior just sat in the back of the room and paid no attention to what was going on in the ward I was perturbed. When a patient went to him with an issue he never even asked what the issue was, instead all he said to the patient was "whatever my staff says goes". It is nice to be supported but all I got out of this remark was that he did not want to be bothered.

A few weeks later he would tell me that he was not going to do my job for me. We went in to a room alone and had a little talk. I flatly told him that I did have an attitude at this place but I was doing my best to do my job. I told him that I would support him as my senior as my job dictated me too, but he had to understand my point of view.

A couple months later I was sent an email moving me to another ward. I went to my senior and asked what this was. He stated that he knew nothing about it. I asked him if he had any issue with me and if he asked for me to be moved off the ward. He denied knowing anything and said he was fine with me working the ward with him. I called my shift supervisor and she told me I was being moved back to my original ward and that it should be considered a good move not a bad thing. I informed her that I was comfortable on the ward, all my stuff was here and that I spoke with my senior and he told me he had no problems with me. My shift supervisor hesitated for a couple minutes then she told me right out that my senior has been down in the supervisor's office for the last three months trying to get me reassigned off the ward. I did not know what to say to that. I knew she was telling me the truth. I gathered my belongings and went to the other ward.

I was more hurt by the fact that he lied with a straight face right to me. He was the one promoted why can't he just tell the truth. I never forgave him for lying to me. I was struggling before to follow his orders now there was just no way. Neither one of us has spoken to the other since I moved off the ward. I laugh inside when I see him. What a coward. If he was straight up with me I would not have had an issue with me moving off his ward. I guess some people never learned anything about integrity.

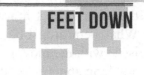

FEET DOWN

JUST LIKE IN THE ARMY when you get the young specialist promoted to sergeant, the new power and control seems to go to their heads, so was the new SRSHTA's. It was like they needed to prove themselves and they were like rats scurrying around to get the one piece of cheese that is out of place. Everyone was on edge over them trying to catch someone doing something wrong so they could write them up to show their power. Maybe this was my problem, but as I told my chief of security I am too old, too tired, and been through too much in life to even worry or even care about them going out of their way to harass people.

You can see that work is getting harder and harder to focus and be in a good spirit here. One night at 2200hrs I was working and I went down the hallway to do our dorm checks of the patients. I did not know it but one of the power seeking SRSHTA went down to get a soda and noticed that I was leaning back in my chair with my feet up. Noticed, what a joke he had to literally go out of his way to look through the window in the door to see me. Well as I was down the hallway he called the ward and told my co-worker to tell me to get my feet off the table. They told him no and for him to do it himself. When I got back from my dorm check my co-worker did not say anything to me about the call. I sat back down grabbed my sudoku book, put my feet up and looked for another number.

About this time the SRSHTA comes on the ward and starts yelling at me from down the hallway at the door, which is a good 70 yards give or take away. I turned around to see who it was and then went back to my book. The entire time he was walking towards me he kept spouting off about supervisors don't want your feet on the furniture. I did tell him I did not care and he kept on. He got next to me and then threatened me for not following his order. I told him he did not give me an order just said the supervisors don't want feet on furniture. He then asked me to put my feet down and I complied. I asked him "What did you come over here just to fuck with me?" He said yes and he kept on counseling me in a hostile voice, until I got tired of it and told him

I was done with my lecture and to go away. He left but soon after I got a call to go to the supervisor's office. When I got there he took me in a room started to counsel me on the incident. I was done talking to him and I told him flat out that I don't mess with him and for him not to fuck with me. I am done talking to you and if you want to talk some more get a union Stewart and I left.

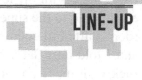

The next evening during line up I was not called off to any ward. I joked to the supervisor;

"If you don't need me I will go home."
"You will sit right there and wait till after the seniors meeting."

SO I SAT THERE DOING my sudoku. Two union Stewarts came down to the line-up room to talk to me. Seems my little comment was taken to heart and I was going to be spoken to about last night. When they sat down and started talking to me I had to ask them what they were talking about and that it did not happen that way. I told my side of the story and they went and spoke with the chief of security. He spoke with the senior in question who stood by his story. Because there was a difference in our stories they held a small gathering after the meeting. I guess before they were just going to walk me out or something.

In the meeting was the chief, two union Stewarts, my shift supervisor, my senior, the senior who I had the issue with and myself. The senior who made the complaint started off. His side of the story was so distorted that I had to chuckle some. Seems his opinion was that he never screamed at me from down the hall, and when he asked me to put my feet down I flatly refused and told him I did not give a fuck about what the supervisors wanted. He went on to say that I was told by the other staff about my feet on the table and that I was the one screaming at him. I listen to his story and I did not interrupt. I took a couple of mental notes on some key areas that were not explained as I believed them to be.

When I started to tell my side of the story I was interrupted right from the start by the senior. I said I quietly listened to your side of the story and that I would like to talk without being interrupted. I explained everything as it happened from me going down to check the dorms and him calling the other staff to tell me to put my feet down, and the fact that they never told me. I stated that he even said to me that he came onto the ward just to fuck with me and that he had to go out of his way to see if my feet were on the table. I said that he started yelling from the minute he walked on the ward, and of course he had to interrupt me again and said he did not say anything until he was next to me. I called him a liar to his face right in front of the chief. I told the chief everything that happened exactly as I remembered it to go even that I said, "I don't give a fuck what the supervisors want". I told the chief that he created this issue by promoting people with a lower score over me and them thinking they could intimate me. I am too old, been through too much in my life, to be treated like this or to be scared of them. I also stated that the other two staff that was on the ward with me was working today and that he could call them down to get their side of the story if he did not believe me.

I was told later by the union Stewarts and by my senior that you could tell that the senior was lying and that I was telling the truth. The chief did not ask to see the other staff and said that he was going to write me up, but he would keep the write up in his desk and if I did not have another issues for a year he would give it back to me and it would not be in my record. I asked the chief what I was being written up for since I felt I did nothing wrong but stand up for myself. The chief stated that I was being written up for arguing with my superiors. I guess he was right I did argue or stand up for me; I guess it is only in the way you look at things. Today I wish I would have not signed the write up and asked for a formal investigation into the situation.

I did have one request before I signed the write up. I requested to be moved to the day shift. The chief asked if I wanted days, and I told him no I did not want days but if I don't get off this 3 to 11 shift with all these new seniors who were promoted over me I will end up losing my job. The chief agreed to me being moved and even gave me three days off before I started the new shift. It was the last time I would be assigned to the 3 to 11 shift.

GOING TO DAYS

I WAS VERY WORRIED ABOUT going to days. I was unsure what kind of a welcome that I would receive. I believed that there was a click going on with the staff at work that golf, play baseball, motorcycle ride, and snowmobile together. I had to prepare myself for the move that I did not want to do, but knew I had to if I wished to keep my job.

When I did finally show up for my day shift I was assigned to a new ward. It seemed all the undesirable staff was all assigned to this one senior there. I just tried to keep as quiet as possible and maybe I could go unnoticed. Surely I was throwing that Hail Mary because there is no way I won't be noticed. My new senior gave me no trouble, no counseling, nothing. He just let me come in and do my job. About the only thing that I could say bothered me was the fact that a staff who came to the facility after me, and was shown some of the ropes by me was this senior's go to staff on the ward. I guess since he has seniority over all the other staff assigned to the ward, he has been on the ward for some time, he was qualified as a trainer for the state, and helped out the senior on the computer he deserved to be his number one guy.

Well I told my new senior that I don't play third string to anyone. Maybe it was me who had the issue. I know that I don't have a middle ground it is either all or nothing. This could be a bad trait or a good trait, depending on your view of things. I was still attempting to do a good job at work. I was still trying to better myself. It is not that I had a issue with this other SHTA. I guess I was just still a lot on edge over the incident on the other shift and of being passed over and not knowing why.

I did get a warm welcome from most of the SHTA's, and a couple SRSHTA about how they thought that I was right with my dealing with the other SRSHTA, and that he has been pushing a lot of my peers around. Rumors went around that the supervisors told the new SRSHTA's to write someone up, so they were all trying to find someone doing something. We all know how rumors go; it is a little truth and a lot of stretching. I thanked everyone who supported me and I just kind of tried to stay out of any spotlight.

Things kind of worked themselves out. I just came to work and did what I always have done. I just was myself and I interacted with the patients like normal. I got a good chuckle two months later when my new senior told me that the supervisors on days congratulated him on straightening me out. He told me he told them he did nothing but treat me with respect and let me do my job. I told him that I was just doing what I always have done but that he should have taken the credit for it anyway.

On the next round of promotions management changed tactics, or as they put it to me later that there was new upper management who changed how the promotions went. First they asked for a letter of intent of interest for all SHTA's. Then they scheduled interviews. During the interview the two supervisors who were conducting it asked a fellow SHTA and myself, who were both union Stewarts, how being a union Stewart would affect us being a senior. Asking us this is totally against the rules and regulations of the agreement between the union and the state for this title.

In March 2007 four SHTAs were promoted one with a score of 95, one with a score of 90, and two with a score of 85. These scores were off the new list that I again scored a 90 on. Again I did not receive an explanation of why I was passed up. I did resign as a union Stewart soon after this. The other SHTA who was asked about how being a union Stewart would affect him being a senior put in a grievance when he was not selected because they mentioned him being a union Stewart. He did win his grievance in arbitration in the year 2012. He won some back pay and his seniority for SRSHTA was back dated, but the facility agreed to this because they were under the impression that he would not be back to work because he was going out on disability for good.

RULE OF THREE / 70.1 TRANSFER

IN 2008, SCORE NOTICES WERE mailed on average, within 90-120 days after the date the exam was given. Your final score will be mailed to you at the same time as the list of passing candidates is established. This list is called the eligible list. Agencies request the eligible list and send out "canvass letters" to enough high scoring eligible to fill their jobs. A canvass letter is an inquiry into your interest in the job and its location, and your availability. Canvass letters are not job offers. If you receive a canvass letter, do not leave your present employment. Do return the canvass letter by the return date if you are interested in the job. If you return the canvass letter late, the agency is not required to consider you for that job. However, your name will remain active for future canvasses. While the law does not require agencies to canvass or conduct interviews, in most cases they do. However, agencies are required to hire from the eligible list according to the **rule of three.**

The eligible list ranks candidates according to their scores. Those with tie scores are given the same rank. The lists are provided to State agencies where the job openings are located. They must follow the rule of three when selecting candidates to interview for a position. The higher your score the better your chances are for getting an interview. Agencies first send out canvass to determine who is interested in the type of appointment at a certain location. Only those who reply on time and say they are interested and who are "reachable" within the rule of three may be appointed. As the list is used to hire people, and as people on the list indicate they are not interested in a position, agencies make their way down the list in score order.

If you are the top scorer you might be considered for the job, but having a high score does not guarantee that you will be hired. All candidates at the highest score are immediately eligible for consideration for appointment. Candidates at lower scores can be considered only when there are fewer than 3 candidates at higher scores. Any candidate's eligibility for appointment depends not only on his or her rank but also how many other candidates are tied at that and higher level ranks.

The following two examples illustrate how this might work.

EXAMPLE ONE:		
SCORE	NUMBER OF CANDIDATES AT THIS SCORE	RANK OF CANDIDATES
100	1	1
95	1	2
90	1	3

In example one above all three candidates of all three scores and ranks are equally eligible to be appointed or reachable.

EXAMPLE TWO:		
SCORE	NUMBER OF CANDIDATES AT THIS SCORE	RANK OF CANDIDATES
100	5	1
95	10	6
90	25	16

In example two above only the 5 candidates at score 100 and rank 1 are eligible for appointment. If however, through hiring or declinations the number of candidates at 100 is reduced to 2, then all 10 candidates at score 95 (rank 6) can also be considered. Only if there were only 2 or fewer candidates at the score of 100 and 95 (ranks 1 and 6) can any of the 10 candidates at the 90 score be considered.

Most eligible lists last for up to four years. However, a list can be superseded by a new list after one year. If you decline a canvass by either letter or telephone, or at the interview, your name may be inactivated for the type of appointment, or agency or location. You may remain eligible for other jobs, however you should ask about the effect of your declination on your future eligibility. If you decline or are unable to accept a job at the time you may later reactivate your name. However, if you receive a permanent appointment from the eligible list, your name will be removed.

A transfer is the movement of a permanent competitive class employee from a position in one title to a position in a different title or from a position in one agency to a position in another agency. Both positions must be within the competitive class. Transfers occur with the consent of the employee after nomination by the appointing agency and the approval of the Department of Civil Service. Approval by the agency from which the employee is transferring is not required in order for the transfer to occur. Generally employees must have had at least one year of permanent service in their current title or at their current salary grade, and the transfer can be to the same or any lower salary grade, but cannot be to a title more than two salary grades (or one M grade) higher than their current title. Employees who are currently serving probation are eligible to transfer. Transfers may not be approved if mandatory reemployment lists exist for the title to which transfer is sought.

There are three different kinds of transfers defined by the Civil Service Law.

1. **Section 70.1-**
   - Allows transfer without further examination from one title to another when a sufficient degree of similarity exists between the minimum qualifications, tests and/or duties of the specific titles involved. The appropriateness of transfer is decided on a title-by-title basis at the request of personnel offices of state agencies. This section of the law also allows employees to transfer to another agency in the same title.

2. **Section 70.4-**
   - Allows transfer to a title which is not similar, but where the employee meets the qualifications for the title. Usually the employee must pass an examination open to the public for the title before transfer can be approved.

3. **Section 52.6-**
   - Allows transfer between administrative titles at the same or similar salary grade. Administrative titles are those involving law, personnel, budgeting, methods and procedures, management, records analysis or administrative research.

Why have rules and regulations if you are going to put loop holes in it for people to manipulate the system to obtain their personnel choice of who gets hired. I mean why have a test? What safe guards does someone have since management is always right? Or should I say management has the right to manage.

It is the answer to all questions. The question I have though is where the line between managing and controlling is.

Manage;

1. To direct or control the use of.
2. To exert control over / to make submissive.
3. To succeed in accomplishing one's purpose: get along.
4. To direct or administer.

Control;

1. To exercise dominating influence or authority over: direct.
2. To regulate or verify by systematic comparison.
3. Authority or ability to regulate, dominate, or direct.
4. A check or restraint.
5. A standard of comparison for comparison for checking experimental results.
6. A set of instruments for operating a machine or vehicle.
7. An organization to direct a space flight.

How can someone like me with all my experiences be passed over and over again year after year and no one has to justify any reason why. I am a retired disabled combat veteran with 24 years of service where I obtained the rank and grade of MSG / E8. I am trained in the Army for SGLI (small group leadership instructor) and have taught ANCOC (advanced non commission officer course), and BNCOC (basic non commission officer course). I have a Top Secret security clearance, and while I was in Iraq I was the S2 NCOIC (intelligence) for our BN. I was in charge of all linguists from recruiting them to assigning them to our companies. I handled all captured equipment, and also ran our BN's detention center where I personally process 385 detainees. I was in charge of all the generator, and their running and maintenance for the entire FOB.

I scored a 90 on both state civil service tests for SRSHTA, and I have nothing but outstanding yearly reviews. Is it too much for me to ask what kind of a reason they had to pass me up or how to better my job performance? What reason could there possible be? How does one expect someone to put forth their best effort if they are ignored or just plain disregarded as if they are just a piece of trash?

Why is it that the facility has changed from their normal hiring routine to use different tactics to get around the eligibility list and get to whom ever they want to promote? What happened to the rule of 3? What good is those tests score if management can just say at a whim that they are doing a 70.1 transfer, and won't be going off the eligibility list? Why can't the person who makes the decision to hire someone just say it was them and not point the finger toward somewhere else? Of course they don't know who did it either. Does anyone ever take ownership for what ever decision they make ever? It's like working with nothing but politicians, all they do is talk yet they rarely say anything.

When does it go from managing to mismanagement? Or better yet how do you prove, or who do you prove to that something is unjust, unfair, or just down right spiteful. Even if the facility's management were right to wonder if I could or could not handle the stress, isn't it discrimination if I am never given the opportunity to try? How can a state facility that trains it staff yearly no that deals with patients daily on emotional issues and how to spot them before they get to the point where someone just says enough and commits suicide, treat one of their own employees like this?

How can this state facility not even speak to me about what I have been through and what I am going through or even if I had any issue that they could help me with? I never ever asked for anything extra then anyone else. All I wanted was fairness to go on with my life and forget about going to Iraq. Even if the facility's management did not notice any signs that I might have been showing of having PTSD, why when I openly asked and looked for help to be just brushed aside by everyone?

Is it not so blunt that you can or can not see it in my story, or the fact that I have proof by emails, and grievances that I felt mattered and to get no answer or the great answer of DENIED, really makes you think you matter or are wanted. How much is enough? How much before someone just gives up, or in my case goes the extra mile to get my questions answered? If it takes standing in front of a judge to get someone to answer my questions then so be it. I deserve to be treated like I am someone. To be treated like this state mental health hospital is treating me is even more frustrating. How can people not see or not try to understand my point of view, my actions, or my moods. The more my frustration grew at work the farther away from reality I went. Which only made my anger grow and I even questioned if I even meant anything to anyone.

Sometimes I wonder how some things I can't remember yet some things are crisp and clear. I feel and live the humiliation, and belittlement that management has bestowed upon me all the time. Sometimes it because of someone I see who was promoted over me or who had a say in my eyes over who got promoted. Sometimes it is because people in positions that most would say have authority over me just not doing their job or trying to push people around just because they can. The fact that I am wrong because I am only a SHTA and they are right just because they are a SRSHTA or higher is just unacceptable to me. I cringe every time I walk into the facility.

The truth is the only thing that management has gotten out of me by not helping me or communicating with me truthfully is an employee who falters on their own work ethics. I now am an employee who does not put forth as much effort as he use to do. I guess it is your opinion whether management has beaten me or not. I don't feel beaten by them, I feel unwanted and I know if they had even a small reason to fire me I would be gone.

It is too bad for them. I could have been one of those leaders who made a difference. Who looked for change for the better? I could have set an example for my peers, and upper management. I could have. I was denied not because of any reason that I know of. I was denied because I stood up for myself. I was denied but they did not win. They lost. They lost all of my devotion and all of my experiences. They lost me, and all they gained was a number. Even less I think. A number can be counted on, and I could care less about any of management's issues. I guess they did beat me after all.

AROUND APRIL 2008 CANVAS LETTERS were sent out to get a new list of potential new SRSHTA's. When the facility received the list after the deadline for the canvas letters there was three 90's. The facility has up to this point used the rule of three. All three of the 90's were from employees in my facility, and management did not want any of them. So if you don't want any of them you have to find a legal way around them. Their first attempt to go around the three of us was to send out new canvas letters, but this time they changed the hours of the job. They posted two different 12-hour jobs with weird hours. They ran into a couple problems with this though.

- All three of us sent back both canvas letters, which meant that the three of us 90's were on each promotion list.
  - o There would be a different list for each canvas letter.
  - o They could of use either lists to hire off of.
  - o They were hoping one of the lists would only have two 90's on it. If say someone did not want those hours and did not send that one canvas letter back.

- The seniors at the facility put in a grievance over the posting.
  - o They should have posted any shift that had different hours, or different days to the seniors already working.

Also in May a 70.1 Transfer Eligibility Letter went out on the facility's Internet asking interested people who qualify to apply.

- o To qualify you have to be within two pay grades of the job title.
- o Have to meet the minimum requirements of the job title.
- o Or be reachable on the civil service promotion list.

The reason for the 70.1 is clear to me that the facility did not want to hire off of the promotional list for this series. Forget that people pay money to take the test and to be placed on the eligibility list. Lets just ignore the eligibility list because we can't get who we want to get. Well interviews were held and they hired two SHTA's who worked at our facility using the 70.1. Both of these SHTA's were on the promotion list one with a score of 85, and the other with a score of 75. That's right I said 75.

INFORMING THE DIRECTOR

I DID NOT KNOW WHERE to turn to too get any kind of an answer. I have tried to talk to all the supervisors, to the chief of security, filed a grievance, all to get no answer on anything. Most people might have given up by now, but not I. I was going to go see a private lawyer to see if I had a case to sue the facility. Being that I was a military man and I understood what the chain of command meant I gave the director of the facility a courtesy email explaining my frustration. I did not ask to speak to him; I just did not want him to get a call from his higher without him having any knowledge of it. Sounds stupid but I felt it was the right thing to do.

Dear Director,

I am sorry that I have to take the time to write to you on this subject, I know you are a busy person and that this issue might seem to be nothing much to you. I believe that as the director of my facility you are ultimately the man responsible for everything that happens here. I am sure that sooner or later that this issue will pass through your desk. I have to believe that it has already but if it has not I wanted to let you know so you would not be caught off guard.

I have been employed here since 2002. The governor activated my National Guard unit and I had to serve a tour of duty in Iraq. Since coming back I have endured many issues, not only here but in my personal life as well. I have found the strength to fight for me and not to give up on everything.

No matter what I do I feel that I cannot be given a fair chance at this facility on any promotions or even the courtesy of a reason why I am being treated so. I have asked in person all of the supervisors as well as the chief himself about what I am doing wrong, what I can do to better myself and my job performance, and why I was never even approached by anyone about being a senior or even the courtesy to say that I was not chosen.

This has created many issues. I find it hard sometimes to even want to try anymore. I cringe when I see certain people. It truly has left me in a dilemma of my integrity and my work habits. I no longer can just sit back and be treated as nothing by the management. I recently put in a grievance on discrimination and hostile work environment, requesting a notarized letter of why I have not been chosen and an apology for being treated this way.

I do not think that I have asked for much from my grievance. I just want to finally know what is this facility's stance on why I am being treated so and how to better myself here. I received my answer on the step 1 grievance . . . DENIED . . . DENIED . . . for 6 years I have been asking why. Just asking why . . . such a simple little question, and the only response I get even after turning in a grievance is DENIED . . . such a nice answer.

I see that no matter what I do or whom I talk to at this facility I will not get a straight answer or be treated with any kind of respect. There for I have been left with no other choice then to seek help elsewhere. Maybe no one in management thinks that I am worthy of a answer. But I know I am worthy of one.

Sincerely

I was a little surprised when the director emailed me back asking for a meeting with the chief and him.

"Can you meet with me and the chief in my office on Wednesday, August 4th at 2 PM? Let me know, thanks."

"I am always willing to talk to you if you have the time . . . Only question I would ask is if I needed a union steward there or not?"

"Your choice entirely, I am open to their attending or not, your call."

"Ok. Thanks for getting back so fast to me . . ."

The meeting was held on August 04 as the director requested and the following is my notes from that meeting.

Notes from the meeting held August 04 2010 in facility director's office.

Present at meeting   . . . . Facility Director
                             . . . . Facility Affirmative Action
                             . . . . Facility Security Chief
                             . . . . My Union Chief Stewart
                             . . . . Myself

Everyone was introduced

I handed everyone a packet full of my yearly reviews, and a list of events up to this point.

A few minutes were given for every one to look over the packet.

The director asked me what was the issue and what was I seeking.

I stated that I was seeking the reason for not being approached about being a senior, and also how I could better my job performance here at this facility. I have been seeking this information since 2005, and I do not seem to be able to get a straight answer from anyone, and that numerous people with a lower test score were promoted over me. I also turned in a grievance, under hostile work environment and discrimination that came back denied on the step 1 process.

The director asked the chief of security what were the job duties of a SRSHTA.

The chief stated job duties of a senior, and the expectations of a Red Dot senior.

The director stated that the facility has the right to use the rule of three and that it has been done in each case.

The chief stated that the last hiring of a senior in the facility used 70.1 and there fore did not go off the list and that the rule of 3 did not apply.

I asked what my issues were since all of my yearly evaluations showed me as more then capable, and that I have nothing negative in my file.

The chief stated that I have not been signing my yearly reviews.

I stated that I have refused to sign my reviews every since I have been passed up for promotions and all of my reviews showed no reason for this.

The director stated that not all areas are covered in the yearly review sheet.

I asked even if there was other areas not covered by the form that I should be counseled by my senior on any part of my job that I is lacking at.

The director asked if my senior was or was not counseling me.

I stated that I wished not to put my senior's work ethics on view. I spoke neither negative nor positive toward my senior. I felt it was best to just remain neutral, as my senior was not present to speak on his own behalf.

The chief stated that he knows that my senior speaks to me on my job performance regularly.

I asked what is the issue with me.

The chief stated that I have replied to some emails and that I have talk negatively throughout the building.

I agreed that I have answered some emails but that I was honest and truthful in them. I also stated that I have talked negatively about not being approached as a senior or given the reason why even after all my attempts to get a straight answer. I asked again why I was not approached about a senior position within the 15 times before I started answering any emails.

The chief stated that my "mental stability would be in question if I was given the job of SRSHTA from all the stress."

I asked the chief what he meant by that and who said that.

The chief then said he had nothing to do with the selection of the new seniors but that he supports the decision made by his supervisors.

I then asked the chief specifically if he had anything to do with the selection of the seniors.

The chief said he had nothing to do with the selection but that he heard that my interview was going good before it went astray.

I stated that I was answering all the questions asked of me and stated to the board "I could answer questions all day by a book answer. I then asked a supervisor why he would want me for a senior and also why he would not me for a senior.

The supervisor replied "the only way I would not select you for the job is if someone was more qualified."

I stated that I was honest and straightforward at the interview.

The director stated that it was a good start and that the chief and my senior would work more closely with me so I can achieve the information that I seek in the future.

Now that the meeting with the director was over, I was even more certain that there was no real justice in the building for me. All I got was we will try and have more conversations in the future with you to try and give you the answers that you seek. Now if I ever heard a cop out that was one. Something someone running for governor would say. You don't answer when confronted; you just push it off on to someone else on another day. That really did nothing to make me feel any better. Why did I even think that seeing the director would change anything?

Maybe if I was given a reason that I could accept. How can you do that when there is not one? Truth is that I don't play softball, golf, motorcycle ride, or even snowmobile with the bigger bosses. I am not part of the click. I am the odd man out. Maybe I was a little rough around the edges. This places runs for people who are rough around the edges.

Worse part is that I knew they would not tell me a reason, because I knew they did not have one. If there was a reason and they gave it to me at least I could work on changing things. Work on conforming into a better leader for them. What a joke. How could the state do this? Is there a place anywhere in the world that is fair to everyone? We all know there is not. After all the only difference from a convict and me is that they got caught. Everyone breaks rules and laws some how or some way.

That is what hurt the most, trying to communicate to those over me who just brushed me aside as if I was a piece of dirt. Most might just sit in the corner where they were swept to. Maybe I was in that corner but I was still sticking out where I could be seen. I still went through the motions of wanting a promotion, even after I knew I would never accept one.

MOVE THAT LOCKER

AS I SAID BEFORE CHANGE always comes, and in this case my SRSHTA was being moved to the woman's ward. He was told that it was only going to be for six months. I laughed at him and told him he would retire on the ward. He was being switched with the SRSHTA who was assigned there. It seems that the woman's ward hardly ever makes it off the ward for any off ward programming, and a very high percentage of all the facilities restraints were happening there.

It is not rocket science what happened when they made the switch. Magically the woman's ward started making it to their entire off ward programming, and the number of restraints dropped sharply. Of course the opposite happened on the ward that we left. If that was not bad enough I had to scold my SRSHTA because he was still doing things for the old ward that the new SRSHTA should have been doing.

"But if I don't do it they will go without, and that is not fair for them."

"I don't care. If you do it he never will, and that is not fair to me or our patients. Maybe someone should make him do his job! You would think they would have noticed the change in both wards."

There is no word to describe someone who always does the extra for no other reason then he can. Someone who makes you feel like you are safe, and like you are a part of the team. I could even say you feel like a part of the family. That was the reason when he asked me if I wanted to stay where I was or move with him to the woman's ward. I told him I did not care where he went I wanted to be there working for / with him.

Of course on the other side is the one who because of his position thinks that they are better then everyone else under them, and they always seem to have to prove it. Don't know if they are proving it to themselves or if they think they are proving it to others. It is my belief that a good leader does not have to show his authority to be in charge.

There is a difference from making a decision because you have to and making one just because you can. Maybe they are trying to make up for something they are lacking. Anyway the SRSHTA who replaced my SRSHTA on my old ward was one of the later. A fucking smuck in my eyes and although today I don't give him the time of day at the time of the switching of the wards I was still listening to and even speaking to him. Not anymore though. I laugh when I see him. If he only knew what a real man was. What a real decision was. I mean a real life changing decision. I bet he is one of those that freezes and can't hold his own when it really counts. One of those leaders that the only way they could be helpful to keeping people safe would be to shoot themselves in the head. Of course I bet he does not have it in him to even do this little task. Who knows maybe if he asked me or even if he did not ask me, I am sure I could spare a bullet, and I am sure I got what it takes.

Well soon after the ward switch the SRSHTA on my old ward called me and told me that I needed to clear out my locker on that ward. First of all he was really rude and loud when he told me this. It was like he was trying to sound important or maybe trying to intimidate me, or something. That was his first mistake. Maybe if he would have spoken to me like a human being I might have gave it at least a little consideration. There is no locker policy in the facility and staffs have lockers all over the building. Hell you work all over the building so it really should not matter where your locker is. I did have my name on two lockers, one had my personnel belongings in and the other one held our shifts cooking equipment. So I cleared out the locker with all the cooking equipment in it.

When this individual noticed that I still had a locker on the ward he approached me in person and told me I needed to clear out the locker. I told him that I cleared out the one and that I planned on keeping this one. "Don't bust my balls." He said, and then he left. Less then an hour later a supervisor came and took me to the side to speak to me. I said, "That did not take long." He laughed with me. I spoke to the supervisor about people having lockers all over the building, and there is no locker policy, and how I thought it was wrong for him to tell me to clear mine out. The supervisor did not tell me to move my locker he asked me to think about it to appease the SRSHTA. Like a good little subordinate I told my supervisor that I would think abut it.

On 4-30-11 I received an e-mail from this supervisor saying that he anticipated me clearing out the locker. I wrote back to him and said that as I recalled our conversation you did not tell me to clear out the locker, and I asked him if he was just acquiring as to if I was going to clear out the locker or if I was going to utilize it. The supervisor wrote back to me saying he would like me to clear it out.

Now maybe this sounds like an order to you but it did not to me. Hell I am surely not a kiss ass and besides no one even asked me if there was a locker on the new ward I was on, which there was none. Of course this is no concern to the SRSHTA all he wants is what he wants and he don't care if it is fair or not. I guess most people would have just moved their locker just for the fact that they did not want any problems. I surely am too stupid to do the simple thing like that.

I then wrote to our Union Stewart and asked if there was a locker policy and if there was could I get a copy of it. I did not receive a e-mail back from him but we spoke in person and we discussed that there was no locker policy in the facility, and that he thought that I was being singled out. A month later I did write to the Chief Union Stewart and requested that the union address the issue for me because the SRSHTA kept telling me over and over again to clear out the locker. I did finally tell him that I was not going to clear out the locker. "We will see" was his comment back to me.

Shortly after this I received a e-mail from the supervisor telling me I was being given a direst order to clear out the locker, and if I did not further actions may be taken. I wrote back and informed him that I have been in contact with the union and that I thought it was unfair for me to be singled out and order to move my locker, and if he planned on doing a facility wide movements of lockers.

Dennis,

I am giving you a direct order to clear out your locker on 201—if you don't follow this direct order, further action may be taken.

Supervisor,

I have been in contact with the union on this issue before and they informed me that there is no policy that states where my locker is. I don't see how it is fair to single me out on where my locker is? Are you prepared to do a facility wide movement on lockers?

I also wrote to the security chief asking for his assistance in the matter. Believe me it took a lot for me to write to him after everything else that has gone on between him and I. I did not expect much help from him but I was giving him the opportunity to let me know his opinion whether it is to ask me to move the locker or to explain to the others that I do not have to move it.

Chief,

Since moving to 601, the SRSHTA on 201 has been telling me to clear out my locker on 201. I did give him the extra locker that had all of my cooking gear in but I kept one there that has my personal belongings in. A racket ball racket, shorts and sneakers, a hat some paperwork and some extra food. I have in the past interacted with patients on the court. I see no reason to move these items to 601 even if I did have a locker there, as I don't see me interacting with the female patients as I did with the males and I still work on the other wards. The locker is in a place where if I needed something I could get it.

I don't understand how I can be ordered to clear my locker out on 201. There is no empty locker on 601 and, even if there was I don't know if I would want to move it. I don't know of any policy on where ones locker is located or on who has the authority to order someone to move out his or her belongings. I have been in contact with the union and they also don't know of any policy.

I am writing to you to clarify to me if there is a policy and if so how do I get a copy of it?

I have forwarded the last message that the supervisor has sent me, where he is threatening me with some further action if I don't. I don't wish to be perceived as ignoring a supervisor but I also feel that this request is beyond the aspects of his authority.

The Chief never responded to my e-mail even though I saw that he opened it. Two days after I sent the e-mail to him a SRSHTA told me that he heard some supervisors, and the Chief in the PCS (personnel control station) office talking and laughing about cutting my lock off the locker and taking my belongings to personnel. My jaw must have dropped a mile. I wish I could say I did not believe what I was hearing, but I did, and it pissed me off to say the least. I mean I just wrote to him and now without the courtesy of any kind of reply the Chief is laughing and making arrangements with the supervisors to cut my lock and move my stuff without telling me. Again the Chief shows his true colors to me. Why did I ever think to even try to get a fair dealing from him? It had to have been my fault. I must have had a brain fart or something.

I immediately called human resources and requested to speak to them. I was invited to come right over to her office. I do not think she was surprised to hear from me. She told me that they did in fact discuss my locker situation, but that she never heard anything about them cutting the lock and removing my belongings. She did say she told them it was not fair to make me move my locker if others who had lockers on other wards then their assigned ward were not asked to move theirs as well. Then she told me that the locker was state property and that I needed to follow a direct order and then make a complaint if I thought I was wronged.

After my meeting with human resources I sent out an e-mail to all concerned in the matter of the locker and informed them that I would move the locker on the up coming weekend as long as the building was calm. As it worked out I did not get to move my locker because there was a situation and I got a broken finger blocking a punch from a patient. I did send out another e-mail stating that I would move the locker at the first available time.

To all concerned

I am sorry I did not empty my locker out on 201 on the weekend as I stated that I would. In case you are unaware during a restraint I block a punch from a patient and it was revealed that I have a broken finger and am out on W/C (workers compensation).

I just wanted to say that I am not refusing to follow this direct order even though I believe it to be unfair and unjust. I will clear out the locker at the first available time that I have.

On 5/23/2011 I wrote to the AA and ask that an official complaint be done about the locker for me.

Dear AA,

I so understand your point on solving things at the lowest level possible. The locker issue may seem like a little thing to you, but I assure you that it is not a little thing to me. The longer I have thought of it since speaking to you the more I am sure that a informal complaint won't be anything that I would be interested in. You told me that no matter what I would not get an apology. I ask you what else is there.

At this time I am requesting that my complaint become an official one . . . As always I anticipate more communication with you on this

On 5/25/2011 at 0904hrs AA responded to me.

Dennis,

I am concerned by what appears to be a misunderstanding of our conversation. Just to clarify, I did not tell you that "no matter what you would not get an apology." When you stated that you wanted a written apology from certain individuals, I informed you that while, I could make your request for an apology known; I am unable to force any individual to offer an apology for a perceived wrong.

During our meeting I encouraged you to meet with your management team in efforts to address situations at the lowest level possible. Throughout the conversation, you vacillated between expressing a willingness to discuss the locker issue informally with management and stating that you did not wish to speak with the Chief at all. By the end of the meeting you agreed to a meeting with me and management to work on improving communication, as well as to find appropriate resolution to your concerns. The department has reviewed your concerns regarding the locker situation and is taking steps to address the issue among all staff.

The Chief, Human Resources, and I would still like an opportunity to meet with you in order to discuss how to move forward in a positive and productive manner. Although not required, we welcome you to invite your union representative to participate in this meeting if that will make you more comfortable. Please advise of your availability, and I will schedule the meeting accordingly.

On 5/25/2011 at 1016hrs I wrote back to her and stated that I would love a meeting and the sooner the better.

On 5/25/2011 at 1022hrs AA responded that she would set up a meeting and if I wanted I could invite my union Chief Stewart to the meeting.

On 5/25/2011 at 1540hrs Chief finally wrote to me

Mr. Williams,

Your concern raises an issue that we will need to take a look at. It has been a long time since we have conducted an inventory of our staff lockers. In an effort to resolve this issue we will look to re-establish the occupancy of all of our staff lockers and make sure that they are clearly marked. I expect that this effort will take place within the next few weeks.

As it stands, each staff member is provided with one locker on the ward to which they are assigned. Historically this practice has allowed for an easy means of managing the location of staff lockers and ensuring that everyone has one. On rare occasions we have had more staff than lockers but I do not believe that to be the case at this point. I appreciate your patience as we move forward with a resolution to this issue.

Please feel free to stop by or send an e-mail if you have further concerns.

Maybe I am just being paranoid, but it seems that the minute that I requested a formal complaint that the Chief wrote to me. She must have called or e-mailed the chief right away that I was requesting an official complaint be filed. So you would think that things would be handled in a timely manner no matter what the out come was. Nope and a month later I again e-mailed the AA to confirm that an official complaint was filed.

Dear AA,

I want to confirm that the complaint of the locker was made an official complaint like I requested on the 23rd of May. I know we talked about doing it informally, but I really think it would be in my best interest to have an official complaint filed and when we come to an agreement it could be closed.

I was looking forward to the meeting that we tried to schedule between us all. Sorry that we could not all find the time together.

Thank you and I look forward to your assistance.

AA responded to me.

Hi Dennis,

As we discussed during our meeting, based on the information you provided, the locker issue does not rise to the level of complaint. You wrote to the department head, which informed you that the department would be addressing this issue across all staff. I did agree to help you work through this informally, and am hoping we can find a mutually agreeable time to meet next week. Did you send Human Resources your dates of availability?

Maybe I did not grasp everything that I discussed with the AA. I know I agreed to a meeting but I did not say anything about dropping my official complaint. Some things are time sensitive. It is better to get it officially recorded somewhere before the time limit becomes the issue to dismiss the issue. Beside things were again dragging and I wanted the issue over with. If an official complaint is made then is there not a time limit on them answering me. They have already proved that they cannot be trusted even if they are in a higher position of authority.

On 6/29/11 AA wrote back to me.

Hi Dennis,

Seems we are having quite a time getting all of our schedules coordinated. Are you available on Wednesday, July 6th at 9:00 AM?

Also, I did check on the progress of the locker situation. Since there will be a lot of movement with the new patient population coming in (the ones we were recently notified about), we are going to wait until all of the moves are completed, then straighten out the lockers.

Regards,

The meeting finally took place on 7/06/2011 in attendance was Human resources, AA, Chief, and myself. I had requested that my SRSHTA be allowed at the meeting but management refused to let him. The main issue as they told me was for the purpose of improving communications between management, and me. I guess in their eyes the locker issue was over. In my eyes that was why we were having the meeting. A little miscommunication here, but either way the meetings surely is a sign of everyone wanting to come to an acceptable solution. Or was it just a cover up again? I mean if they were going to be truthful in anything why it is I could not have my SRSHTA there? The meeting seemed to start off in a good direction. Not too far into it the Chief brought up two issues.

The first was that he had heard that I was bringing in and giving stuff to the patients. I explained to the Chief that I did buy with my own money some dirt and flower seeds and I did have a afternoon of planting flowers with the patients on the ward on mother's day. I also had brought in a few small pieces of candy / candy bars that I gave away as the winning to the bingo games that I play with the patients on the ward. I also explained that I had permission from the treatment team to do both of these. The Chief asked for proof of having permission. I told him I use to have it in my e-mail but even if I did not he could ask them since they were in the building. I was told by the Chief that I was not to bring anything else into the facility for any patient for any reason and if he heard of me giving just a piece of candy to a patient that it would be dealt with.

The second comment was that a Union Stewart stated to him that when I spoke to them they had told me that I was being insubordinate. I told the Chief that I did not believe this and he told me that he had a written statement from the Union Stewart in his office.

I did get my defensives up after this comment and I came right out and stated that I thought he was trying to intimate me. His response to me was that he had other options he could have taken and if he wanted to intimate me we would not be having this conversation.

I then told the Chief that he did not have to talk to me at all. After all he is three echelons above me and I got nothing more to say to someone who never does what he says. As a matter of fact you don't even have to give me a hello when you see me in the building.

I then asked the AA and the Human Resources what they thought of the conversation. They both told me that they felt that the Chief was not trying to intimate me and that he was just trying to work out our communication issues like I have been asking for the last five years. I told them I was done with the meeting at that I did not want to have another one.

I did drop into Human Resources later before the end of my shift. She told me that she thought that the Chief was just trying to show that he could have taken a different approach to the situations. I did say to her that I would have another meeting as long as it was taped and I got a copy of it. She flatly refused and asked me why. I said why not you tape interrogations of staff and that I was tired of thinking I heard something and then to be told later that it was never said or that someone else said it. I want to be able to listen to the conversation when I am not so tense and have a better chance of understanding what everyone is trying to say. I was told that it would never be taped and I said then I will never have another one.

After the meeting I wrote an e-mail to my Chief Union Sector Stewart and asked him about the comment that the Chief made and also if he did make and sign a statement like that. He was the only one I spoke to on the issue so it had to be him.

Chief Union Sector Stewart,

I am a little confused about a meeting I had this morning with the Chief, Human Resources, and AA. The Chief stated that a union official made a statement that they told me I was close to or was being insubordinate on the locker issue. As you are the only one I have spoken to from the union on this issue. I wrote to you about a policy but we spoke in person before you could reply and we discussed about us believing that there was not a policy.

I don't believe that I was insubordinate or was even close to it and I surely don't remember you telling me that. I am seeking your opinion on this issue, and if you did write a statement could you tell me what you wrote. Thanks

The Chief Union Sector Stewart wrote back to me:

Dennis,

I think that you know that I would not say anything like that. I don't know and I don't think that the regional vice-president would say such a thing. I did not write anything at all. I have and always will be honest with everyone I help represent in the union. The only thing that we talked about in regards to the lockers is that I thought it was not fair to single you out and that if that is the case management should have everyone move their lockers to their wards if they haven't done so. I recommend that if you do meet with the Chief or human Resources or anyone in administration to talk about policy/procedure or disciplinary matters that you have some union representative with you so that this does not happen.

To which I responded to him:

Chief Union Sector Stewart,

Please don't take offense to me asking. That was not my intentions. As I said you were the only union person I spoke to and the Chief did state that he had a statement from a union representative stating that they spoke to me about being insubordinate on the locker issue. I wrote to you because I did not believe what he said and I wanted to be truthful and honest and make sure that no rumors are spread either way.

We both know what a hard and tiring job of being a union Stewart is, especially in this place. I wrote to you because I do respect you and did not believe that you would have written something like that. Maybe the Chief was just trying to scare me . . . I don't know. I do know that for me to approach you on any issue at all means that I do respect you as a union representative. I know that I am in a bad place with management in the SHTA series here. I don't have any idea of how to fix it. I love my job but hate being treated as I am . . .

Once again thank you for all your help in the past and the future. I would and will still seek you out if I need some help or guidance. There is no greater honor for a man to give then to be able to place his life in another, and that is how I feel I am doing when I come to you, because it is my livelihood . . . it is my life . . .

thanks again

The Chief Union Sector Stewart wrote back to me:

Hey Buddy no offense taken at all if anything I am upset that they would say something like that to you. Maybe they are trying to ruin my credibility with my fellow members who know. Either way the only people that I spoke with about your situation is the Chief, Human resources, and the Regional vice-president . . . And I agree . . . it is a tough environment that we work in. Constantly finding ways to keep peace among our patients/inmates staying in constant good relations with them yet provide structure and enforcing rules . . . all while we experience anger physical harm and threats towards us and at times our families . . . we experience situations that directly affect our psyche and emotional/physical well being everyday that the average person could not handle or be a witness to without giving in or shake their head in disbelief. We go home to our families at times with scars bruise and broken bones . . . but we as SHTA's continually push our reset button and try to put everything behind us and carry on . . . making sure that we try to work with a clear head and keep order within our wards. Not easy at all . . . one day we are being spit at . . . assaulted . . . verbally and physically threatened . . . the next day we are shaking hands and laughing with the same person . . . who or what other job do you ever experience such a emotional roller coaster? This Job is not for the weak hearted or minded! But we have people who seem to think that we have it easy . . . that we are comp abusers . . . the problems of the facility . . . that we are too aggressive with the patients as if we instigate red dots . . . That "PMCS" is the key to solving all situations . . . During my time as Chief Sector Steward I hope to bring some respect to our title, bring unity among us and advertise to our facility and higher as to the conditions we work in . . . I'm here for people like you Joe who put in their time not only for our country but also for our work place and fellow co workers. Once upon a time in this country we awarded men and women like you who have a history of leadership and dedication to this country and work place with positions that continued to thrive and take advantage of their proven leadership skills and dedication . . . We used to reward people of character and integrity . . . I hope that we get their again Joe. Thanks buddy and stay strong and focused.

On 7/9/2011 I wrote to all concerned that I had cleared out the locker. The AA asked me if I got a locker on my current ward and if not to let her know. So I wrote back to her.

AA,

No! I did not get a locker on my current ward. What was I to do? I don't agree with the way that the Chief or the supervisor handled this issue. I did not like the Chief's comment about having a statement from a union official where they told me I was close to being insubordinate. To me it was the chief trying to intimate me even though Human Resources said she did not think so. Cold hard truth is that if I don't move the locker I am wrong for not following a direct order. There never was a locker policy and there never will be. Saying we will wait till something else happens is a cop out. I got nothing else to say to any one in the facility on this issue. If I am told to move my locker again I think I just might not have one.

AA wrote me back:

Dennis,

I don't think the Chief was trying to intimidate you. I do think he was trying to demonstrate that he wants to work with you and not just jump to the most extreme course of action even if he feels there is justification to do so. Also, during our meeting, the Chief said that we would hold off on the locker situation until after the new patients arrived because that was going to create a lot of movement. To my understanding, this included the request for you to move your locker. However, since you have already done so, you should have a locker on your ward. I will follow-up on this.

Regards,

The Chief responded to my e-mail of moving my locker also:

Dennis,

Did you find a locker on 601?

To which I responded to the Chief:

No.

The Chief then ask me in a e-mail:

Are you occupying a locker anywhere else in the building?

To which I replied to him:

Yes,

There were no lockers on 601 as you can confer with the SRSHTA assigned there on this. I found an empty locker on 302. A side note the locker on 201 that was so desperately needed for staff remains unused at this time.

On 7/26/2011 the AA wrote to me:

Dennis,

During our meeting on July 6, 2011 with Human Resources and the Chief, we offered to meet with you on a regular short-term basis in order to discuss/

address any concerns you may have in attempts to improve communication and the work environment. We believe that meeting once per month over the next three months might be helpful. At the time, you declined the offer, so we asked you to think about it. Since some time has passed, I wanted to check back to see whether you have reconsidered our offer.

Also, when we discussed bringing items in for patients, you stated that you had received permission from your Senior and/or the Treatment Team. You indicated that this was confirmed with those individuals via e-mail. Chief asked if you would provide copies of those e-mails to him, so that he could follow-up to make sure that everyone is on the same page about the safety and security risk this poses and so that he can ensure that everyone is aware of the proper protocol. Please let me know whether you had an opportunity to send those e-mails to him.

Again, our goal is to work together in a positive and productive manner.

On 7/27/ 2011 I wrote back to AA:

AA,

First off as I stated in the meeting if you have a issue that I have done something on my own you should contact my immediate SRSHTA. Yes the treatment team gave me permission and knew of the seeds and dirt that I brought in. Yes I am working with the team to do more stuff with the ward, and anything that they receive for prizes is given to me through the recreation people and through my SRSHTA. My SRSHTA is in the building and I am sure the treatment team can't be too hard to reach. I don't have any emails as I deleted them. As far as I am concerned this is a dead issue.

I felt Chief was trying to intimate me in the meeting when he first brings up the issue of saying someone said I was bringing things in for the patients, then he says that I was told by a union official that I was being insubordinate on this issue, when I said I did not believe him he said he had a written statement. I found this very disturbing, for either the Chief was trying to scare / intimate me or a union official is not supporting me when I seek help and guidance from them. I will try to be fair and give Chief the benefit of the doubt. Give me a copy of the statement from the union official that says they told me I was being insubordinate, and I will apology to him and then I can approach the union on it.

To say that everyone is working together I disagree. No one else has been asked / ordered to move their lockers. There is no locker policy and there never will be. I know my SRSHTA approached the other SRSHTA on the locker issue and how he could get all the lockers he needed without bothering me but he was ignored. I was singled out, and when I sought help I was ignored. I don't know how else to look at it.

Yes I did agree to this meeting and as I have said to both you and Human resources in the past, that all I wish for is that I be treated fairly and honestly. Even though both you and Human Resources said to me that you both thought Chief was trying to show that he could of handled things differently if he wished. I did not see it that way. We had the meeting to discuss the locker issue. When I tried to bring up issues that you say happened in the past everyone wants to say that it is in the past and to just let the lawyers handle it and to move forward.

I am sorry if I am not the normal employee in this building . . . I am sorry I feel like I have the right to know why I have been passed up. I am sorry that I want to know how to better myself in the facility. I am sorry that I stand my ground. These qualities got me far in the service. Now all I get is resentment from management at work for these actions.

I have let the past behind me. I am ok with letting the legal system handle my concerns about being treated unfairly / discriminated against in the facility. All I want is to be left alone and stopped being singled out. You will see by my latest complaints that this has not happened. The locker issue was never an issue about just the locker no it was an issue with people thinking that they can push me around just because . . .

I do wait to see how the retaliation complaints go, as I also await for the statement on how I was told by the union official that I was insubordinate.

As far as another meeting goes . . . As long as I am spoken to honestly, straightforward and without hostility I have no problem with any meeting. I will agree to more meeting as management thinks is necessary. Though I don't see why my immediate SRSHTA is not allowed in these meetings. After all would he not be the one to say whether my attitude shows any negativity toward me doing my job or toward the patients?

On 7/27/2011 the AA wrote to me:

Dennis,

There is a lot here, so I am going to try to respond as succinctly as possible and number my responses, so I don't lose track.

1) During the meeting, you said that you were not sure if you had the e-mails from your SRSHTA or the treatment team because you delete a lot of stuff, but you did agree to check and get back to us, so I was just following up.

2) I don't believe the Chief was trying to intimidate you. He was asking you about something that was brought to his attention in a non-accusatory manner. I do believe his intent was to find out what happened, so he could address it properly, as well as to make sure that you understood that he would not be ok with anyone bringing in personally-purchased items for patients. I believe he acknowledged that lots of things were permitted in the past, but that we now operate under different mandates and laws.

3) As far as a statement by a union official, you will have to address that with the Chief and/or your union representative, but again, the intent of our meeting was about working together, not intimidating anyone.

4) I disagree that you were not provided with assistance when you sought help, I feel as both Human resources and I were very responsive and supportive in helping arrange the meeting. The Chief also expressed a willingness to meet with us regularly to help keep things on track for you. As we explained in the meeting, we were notified of new incoming patients, which would result in wide-spread moves. The Chief informed you in the meeting that no one (this included you) would be required to move their locker until after that occurred. He then asked whether you had experienced any negative ramifications for not moving the locker. You stated, "No." Even so, you moved your locker after our meeting. Joe, you did not have to do that, we told you we put the project on hold. Nonetheless, after you notified us that you moved it, we made arrangements to get you a locker on your current ward.

5) There is a whole lot there that we have discussed on numerous occasions, and I can only reiterate that we want to work with you. As far as the meetings go, this really is not about what management thinks is necessary, it is about the fact that you have repeatedly expressed concerns over the way you feel you are being treated or the way certain situations are handled. We are trying to give you a more direct access to address issues and help foster a positive work environment. Of course, this will only work as a team effort.

On 7/30/ 2011 I wrote to the Chief:

Chief,

I respectfully request a copy of the written statement that you said you had of the union official saying that they spoke to me and told me that I was being insubordinate about the locker issue.

I am requesting this statement so that I can bring the matter up with the union steward that wrote it.

On 8/2/2011 the Chief wrote back to me:

Dennis,

I never said that I had received a statement from a union rep. I did say that I had the impression that the union may have shared that thought with you.

On 8/2/2011 I wrote to Human Resources:

Human resources,

I asked the Chief for the statement that he said he had from a union steward during our meeting and this is the reply that I got.

- I never said that I had received a statement from a union rep. I did say that I had the impression that the union may have shared that thought with you.

Now I ask you. How can you expect me to honestly not worry about myself and my livelihood here when all I get is lies, and deception? If the Chief was not trying to intimate me then he should have the statement that he stated he had. If he lied then how anyone can say that he was not trying to push me around?

How can I be mistaken? Did you hear him say this? First he said a union official told him they told me I was told by them that I was being insubordinate, and when I said I did not believe him he said well I have a written statement that says otherwise.

Through out this entire locker situation, management never involved my immediate supervisor. I did keep him informed of all events. In the beginning he went to the other SRSHTA and gave him a suggestion that would solve his issues of having enough lockers for the ward without having me move my locker, but he was ignored.

As of August 2012 there still is not a policy on lockers. Just to clarify things there is not a locker policy. There never has been a locker policy. There will never be a locker policy.

ALLIGATIONS

I WAS TRYING TO LET the locker situation behind me when I responded to a silent dot on ward 201. I was instructed by the SRSHTA (the same one who ordered me to move my locker), to go into the dayroom and have another SHTA come out to the side room. I followed the instructions without hesitation or comment. When I instructed the other SHTA as to the SRSHTA's request he asked me "why? Wasn't I good enough for him?" He did not understand why he was wanted or why I was not wanted out there.

In the dayroom two patients approached me and asked if they could speak to me. Both patients wanted to inform me that the SRSHTA and another SHTA were talking bad about me loudly in the dayroom. They were trying to get another SHTA to make a complaint about me harassing him earlier in the day by the elevators. I did see the SHTA by the elevators and I did speak to him as I always do in a joking manner. He was upset with me over a grievance that I had put in and how it might affect him and his job assignment. I went to speak to this SHTA about the issue of them wanting him to make a complaint against me, and he told me that he did not want to get caught up in their affairs, and that both of them were upset with me over the grievance and the locker issue.

I could not believe what I was being told. I mean I can see the reason for both of them to be a little displeased with me. It should not have been me that they were upset with after all I was just trying to make sure everyone was being treated the same across the board. Now this SHTA has refuses to speak to me and he even slams doors in my face. He goes out of his way to make sure I know what he is doing. You would think that this would have passed, but it continues today. The bigger issue to me was of the SRSHTA. He is upper management, and having him trying to convince my fellow co-workers into making false allegations against me, is both unprofessional and unforgivable to me. After all it is his job to defuse situations and not to make things worse. This is against every aspect of being a good leader and surely can not support any policy. Anyone has the right to make a complaint without the worry of any negative repercussions. Surely this falls right into that category of black and white, how can one not see that?

I called over to Human Resources and explained what I had learned, they asked for a statement about the incident.

SWORN STATEMENT

I DENNIS, J. WILLIAMS, WANT TO MAKE THE FOLLOWING STATEMENT UNDER OATH.

I RESPONDED TO A SILENT DOT ON WARD 201 AROUND 1200hrs. ON 07/15/2011. I WAS INSTRUCTED BY SRSHTA xxxxx xxxxx TO GO INTO

THE DAYROOM AND HAVE SHTA xxxxx xxxxx COME OUT TO THE SIDE ROOM WHERE SRSHTA xxxxx xxxxx, SHTA xxxxxx xxxxx, AND TEAM LEADER xxx xxxxxx WERE STANDING IN FRONT OF THE SIDE ROOM. I FOLLOWED SRSHTA xxxxxxx'S REQUEST WITH OUT HESITATION OR COMMENT. WHEN I INSTRUCTED xxxxx xxxxx THAT HE WAS WANTED OUT IN THE HALLWAY HE MADE A COMMENT THAT HE DID NOT UNDERSTAND WHY HE WAS WANTED, OR WHY I WAS NOT WANTED OUT THERE.

IN THE DAYROOM PATIENTS xxxx xxxxxxx, AND xxxxxxxx xxxxxxxxx APPROACHED ME AND ASK IF THEY COULD SPEAK TO ME. BOTH PATIENTS WANTED TO INFORM ME THAT SRSHTA xxxxx xxxxx AND SHTA xxxxxx xxxxx WERE TALKING ABOUT ME IN A NEGATIVE WAY LOUDLY IN THE DAYROOM, AND THAT THEY WERE TRYING TO GET SHTA xxx xxxxxxx TO MAKE A COMPLAINT ABOUT ME HARASSING HIM EARLIER IN THE DAY BY THE ELEVATORS.

I DID SEE SHTA xxx xxxxxx BY THE ELEVATORS AND I SPOKE TO HIM AS I ALWAYS DO IN A JOKING MANNER. HE INFORMED ME THAT HE WANTED ME TO KEEP A DISTANCE FROM HIM BECAUSE HE WAS UPSET OVER THE GRIEVENCE THAT I PUT IN AND HOW IT MIGHT AFFECT HIM.

I LATER SPOKE TO SHTA xxx xxxxxxxx ABOUT SHTA xxxxx AND SRSHTA xxxxx AND THE ISSUE OF THEM WANTING HIM TOO MAKE A COMPLAINT AGAINST ME. xxx STATED TO ME THAT HE DID NOT WANT TO GET CAUGHT UP IN xxxxxx xxxxx'S AFFAIRS, AND THAT SHTA xxxxxx xxxxx WAS UPSET WITH ME BECAUSE OF THE GRIEVENCE.

SHTA xxxxxx xxxxx HAS REFUSED TO SPEAK TO ME AND IT IS MY BELIEF THAT HE IS TRYING TO GET BACKAT ME FOR THE GRIEVENCE THAT I TURNED IN ABOUT EVERY OTHER WEEKEND SCHEDULE.

I CAN UNDERSTAND SHTA xxxxxx xxxxx BEING UPSET AND MAYBE EVEN A LITTLE MAD BUT SRSHTA xxxxx xxxxxx AS A SENIOR SHOULD BE DEFUSSING SITUATIONS AND NOT TRYING TO INSIGHT STAFF AGAINST ME.

I FEEL AS IF SRSHTA xxxxx xxxxx IS TRYING TO GET BACK AT ME FOR MY REFUSAL TO MOVE MY LOCKER OFF OF WARD 201 WHEN HE TOLD ME TO DO SO.

AFFIDAVIT

I, DENNIS J. WILLIAMS, HAVE READ OR HAVE HAD READ TO ME THIS STATEMENT AND FULLY UNDERSTAND THE CONTENTS OF THE ENTIRE STATEMENT MADE BY ME. THE STATEMENT IS TRUE. I HAVE INITIALED ALL CORRECTIONS AND HAVE INITIALED THE BOTTOM OF EACH PAGE CONTAINING THE STATEMENT. I HAVE MADE THIS STATEMENT FREELY WITHOUT HOPE OF BENEFIT OR REWARD, WITHOUT THREAT

OR PUNISHMENT, AND WITHOUT COERCION, UNLAWFUL INFLUENCE OR UNLAWFUL INDUCEMENT.

Besides giving HR a statement I also filed a complaint of retaliation through AA.

7/24/2011

AA

I slipped two envelopes under your door that I wish to have processed. One is the paper work for a complaint on SRSHTA Xxxxx Xxxxxx, and the other is the paperwork for a complaint against SHTA Xxxxxx Xxxxx, dealing with the retaliation incident that happened on 7-15-2011.

Also. In our meeting Chief said he had a written statement from a union official that said they spoke to me on being insubordinate. I would like to give Chief the benefit of the doubt and believe that he has such a statement. I would like a copy of this statement so that I could bring the issue up with the union. Would you assist me in getting a copy?

Now this was not my first dealing or filing of a complaint through the AA personnel at the facility. So far all she has been concerned with is trying to make my future in the facility a little more comfortable. Maybe, just maybe she looking out for my best interest. I don't think so but let's give her the benefit of the doubt. Now we have a cut and dry case of my co-workers trying to retaliate against me for my filing complaints against them. This must fall into her realm because AA deals with the following issues in the work place:

1. COLOR
2. NATIONAL ORIGIN
3. CREED
4. AGE
5. SEX
6. MARITAL STATUS
7. RELIGION
8. RETALIATION
9. DISABILITY
10. ARREST RECORD
11. CRIMINAL RECORD
12. SEXUAL ORIENTATION
13. VIETNAM ERA VET. STATUS

I waited for a reply from the AA department about my complaints of retaliation. When November came around and I still have not heard anything I called and spoke to the AA personnel. I was shocked at her response to me that it did not fall into her area and that she had sent the complaint to the HR department. How the hell did it not fall into her department, it is a flat out case of retaliation and I even sent her eight witnesses who could back up my complaint? So I called over to HR and asked about my complaint.

On 11/23/2011 I received a email from HR about my complaint.

Hi Dennis,—

You had filed a complaint with AA on 7/23/11 which were then referred to me for action. The complaints were reviewed and dealt with appropriately.

Again I felt as if I was not getting a fair deal. Not only did the AA not deal with the retaliation complaint instead they sent it to the HR department, where a ruling was made (so the email stated) yet none of the witnesses that I sent were ever spoken to. Of course I am not entitled to know what if any disciplinary actions were taken, but the fact that none of the witness of the retaliation complaint were never spoken to makes me believe that management has just swept my complaint under the rug again.

I do acknowledge that management or should we say HR sent me a email stating they dealt with the retaliation issue but how does that solve any of my concerns if:

- They never spoke to any of the witnesses.
- No one has apologized to me, or even spoken to me about my concerns.
- Management has not made sure that I feel comfortable or safe working around them.

I did get management's position in writing from one of my grievances on why I was passed up for promotion over and over again:

Management's position:

Management is aware of Mr. William's standing on the Civil Service list. Each time an appointment has been made, he has been given fair-minded consideration. It should be noted that an applicant's standing on the Civil Service list does not entitle the applicant to a promotion; it merely places that applicant on a list for consideration. Many factors are taken into consideration when an appointment is made. Management has the right to select who they feel is the best person for the position as long as they make the appointment in accordance with the Civil Service Laws, which was done in this case.

Funny it is now the beginning of the year 2013, and I still have yet to be told any reason. As always just push things under the rug so they are not in sight. Maybe they will be forgotten about. Management might have wished for this from me but I have not or will not ever forget about or stop acquiring into why I have been passed over time after time, year after year, and never received any reason why.

ADMINISTRATIVE LEAVE

I REMEMBER THE DAY OF December 9th very well; I went human resources for a grievance hearing. When I got in the room I made a joke about there being a party because of all the people who were in the room around the table. Of course I got no reply from anyone nor was one expected. I took my seat and the normal grievance proceedings took place. When the hearing was done and we all were getting up to leave I was asked to stay after the other grievant left.

The Human Resources member opened a folder and began to read:

Dear Mr. Williams:

This is to inform you that effective **immediately** you are being placed on Administrative Leave with Pay. You will remain on that status until further notice. You are directed to remain off the grounds of this facility and have no contact with any of the employees here without specific approval from the Human Resource Management Office.

At this time, I am requiring you to return your New York State issued identification badges, as well as any other state-issued property that you may have in your possession. Failure to do so may result in criminal charges being brought against you.

You are further directed to contact Human Resources Office daily (Monday-Friday) between the hours of 9:am-11:am.

After the statement was read to me I asked why I was being placed on Administered Leave and all I was told was that it was a serious matter and that it warranted it. I then asked about talking to my girlfriend who works there also, and I was told that I would get into trouble if I did not follow the directions given and that it was ill advised to communicate with anyone who works for our organization including her. I did get very frustrated, especially since I had no idea as to what the issue was. I stood up and stated "why don't you all stop fucking with me and just go ahead and fire me and get it over with." I gave them my badges and left the room. I waited in the waiting room for my personnel belongings to be brought to me, and then I was escorted off the property. Later I learned that there was a rumor running through the building of me flipping out by screaming and throwing chairs around at the grievance committee. It is so nice to know what people think of you sometimes.

I received a notice in the mail certified telling me of my personnel status change. This is standard procedure that is done when ever there is a change in your status. The only issue I had with this was that it stated that I was placed on Administrative Leave with Pay under Disciplinary Suspension. Disciplinary Suspension, hell I had no idea what was going on how they could say it was for disciplinary reasons. Guess I am guilty before proven innocent or in this case before, I even know what is going on. Fairness is so great in the work place.

I followed most of the directions that they gave me. I called the facility every morning Monday to Friday and reported in. I found that my e-mail address for the organization was shut off. I refrained from talking to anyone from work with the exception of my girlfriend. How can an employer even dare to tell you that you can't interact with your lover? I mean I can see if they tell you not to touch one another while you are working but to flatly come out and tell you that you can't have any interactions with someone and not tell you their reasoning are just unacceptable to me. After all who do they think they are the armed forces or what?

I spent a week wondering why I was placed on Administrative Leave. Even though I was on paid leave I was still very upset, and my mind was going over everything that it could think of for them to do this to me. The fact that I could not think of anything just made things worse in my mind. The wondering stopped when the New York State Police called me, and asked me to come down to the station so I could answer some questions. I told him I would come down but I wanted to know if I was being arrested, and if I needed someone to drop me off so my car did not get towed. He told me I was not being arrested and that he just wanted to ask me some questions. I then asked what it was about because I spent the last week worrying about the reason why I was placed on administrative leave. The New York State Police Inspector told me it was for a complaint about a patient. This shocked me and also calmed my nerves, after all I would know if I did or did not do anything with, or for a patient that was against policy.

When I got into the interrogation room with the inspector he asked me if I remembered a certain patient. The name was familiar and after he started telling me some of the details I remember exactly who he was talking about. I started to laugh when he was telling me what I was there for. I asked the investigator why I was out of work if this was what was going on. He told me that he had nothing to do with facility policy and that it was them who took me out of work and it had nothing to do with the State Troopers investigation.

Now it is not uncommon for a patient to make a complaint against a staff member in the facility. Most times it is unjustified and they are doing it just to get the staff in trouble. They seem to cherish the fact that they have the ability to make a change to something, whether it is in the reassignment, or firing of a staff. It comes with the job and all the staff are aware of this. The patients / inmates have nothing but time to ponder what to do or what to say to accomplish what they have set their minds on. If they are trying to get a staff member to do or get something for them and they don't get it them might hold a grudge. If they do hold a grudge they will never forget and may even leave to another facility and it may be years later, and the staff won't remember it and then BAM! You won't even see the assault coming.

I can only speculate as to why this certain individual did as they did. I am sure that they were looking to either get something whether it is in their placement or the fact that when she was here I did something that she did not like and has focused on it. The fact that she did what she did really did not bother me, because as I said it comes with the job. The fact that I was placed on administrative leave because of it is unheard of. I mean I can see moving me off the ward so she would not have to interact with me, but she was no longer in the facility. That is right I said she was not even in the facility. No one has ever been placed on administrative leave for a complaint like this, not even if the patient was still in the building. So how can they justify placing me on the administrative leave? Your guess is as good as mine, but all I can think of is the problems that I have in communicating with upper management in the past and that this was a way of them getting back at me.

I guess you are wondering what the complaint was? Well first let me say that there are no secrets in the facility. People always talk and the inmates are always listening. Hell they can tell you who drives what car, what color, what year even where it is parked on almost any given day. They live their lives through staff's stories. You would be surprised as to how much information that is known about every staff. This information will be used against you if they can.

Ok let's get back to the complaint. I was told by the New York State Police Investigator that a former patient had made an allegation against me when she got to her new prison. She claimed that she and I had sex four times. Three times in the patient's bathroom and once in the ping pong room. She did not claim I raped her but rather said in was consensual sex. She told them her and I are close and that I had three kids.

The investigator asked me if I knew who she was and I said yes I remember her well. He wanted to know how much I remembered about her before he told me any more. Then he stopped in mid sentence. Up to this point I was care free and laughing and joking with the investigator. He told me he had to read me my rights.

1. You have the right to remain silent.
2. Anything you say can and will be used against you in a court of law.
3. You have the right to an attorney.
4. If you cannot afford an attorney, one will be appointed for you.

Then I told him that I knew that she was angry with her boy friend, because she found out in prison that she had been infected by the HIV / Aids virus, and when she called him to tell him he told her that he had the disease for over five years. A real shocker I bet, especially since they have a son together.

"So you knew she had aids? Has anyone ever had any sexual interactions with the patients? Why would you have sex with her if you knew she was positive for HIV?" The investigator asked.

"I wish I could say that something like that has never happened, but it happens more often then one might think. I have never had any sexual contact with any facility patient."

"Why one would chose to have sexual contact with a patient, and do you think they deserve a second chance?"

"Who knows there is different reasons I guess, maybe it is a control thing, maybe it is true love, and no anyone who has any type of inappropriate contact with a patient should not be given a second chance. I mean if someone killed someone would you give them a second chance?"

I had to laugh at the "ping pong" room. I told him we have a game room where there is a ping pong table but when we are there the room is full of the entire ward, but I have played racket ball on occasion with some of the female patients. Of course he asked if I was ever alone in the racket ball room as well.

"I am never alone with a female patient at any time. There is always a female staff with-in eye distance. When we are in the gym there is always staff right outside the window of the racket ball court if I go inside and play whether it is a male or a female patient."

"She stated that you had sex with her when you took her to the bathroom. How do you take a female to the bathroom?"

"I do take females to the bathroom, but I never go into the bathroom, I stand at the door. When ever a female has to be watched closer a female staff will take them inside the bathroom."

He then asked me some pretty straight forward questions about who I work with and how the ward runs on a daily basis. We actually or should I say I actually had a good time, laughing and joking as I was talking with him about everything. He asked me about this and I told him the last week I was concerned about the facilities reason for walking me out but now I think it is a joke.

We finished up and he asked me if I would take a lie detector test, and of course I said I would. He explained a little on this test and then he finished up by telling me what was going to happen now. He said that my co-workers would be questioned and then he would go down to speak to her to see if she stands by her story. He wanted to know the results of the lie-detector test when he went down to see her. He also said that her side of the story did not make as much sense as mine and that her story has changed a little here and there and he wanted to speak with her to see if she would drop the complaint.

I left feeling good. I did not know when I would do the lie detector test but I did jokingly say I wanted it after Christmas. After all I now have it off with pay. He laughed with me and told me that he had nothing to do with the test that they have specific investigators who do them, and that I will get a call when they have it scheduled. I thanked him and left.

Of course my girl-friend was all worried about what went on. She did not understand why some of the things were said and done, and of course she made comments about not talking about your business at work I told her to expect a phone call to be questioned. That phone call never came though.

So I went on with my daily routine, calling in every morning and checking in with the secretary. This went on until December 23rd when I was told that I was off of administrative leave and that I was to report to work starting tomorrow on my normal daily schedule. This was very nice of them to let me come back the day before Christmas. I was not happy. There was no way I was going to work on Christmas. I had done a bunch of swaps that were no longer any good, and I have custody of two of my three girls whose mother has told me she does not want them for Christmas. There was no way I was going in.

I waited until nine o'clock that night and I called the supervisors office. I asked the supervisor if he knew I was cleared to report back to work in the morning, and he said he did. I then said I was calling in sick for three day on family sick leave. He said ok and I hung up. I did not care what anyone said and if the facility was going to LWOP (leave without pay) me, I wanted to make sure I called in well before the one hour deadline.

After Christmas I went back to work. I did not know what to expect but I figured that things would be all ready for me. Of course that is asking too much. I had no identifications badges, and my e-mail account was still blocked by the facility. They sent me right back to the woman's ward, without a word. Funny I can't work because it is such a rotten thing that warranted me being walked out of the job but I can just come back with no counseling, no badges, or access to the internet. Surely I was fine and I did not have anything to worry about!

I worked for about five weeks before my old SRSHTA asked me about an e-mail that he sent me and then noticed I did not have my badge and said something to me. I laughed and told him about my e-mail also. He asked why I did not say anything and I told him it was because I was too stupid to understand what I should or should not do. This was my answer to any questions that management asked me about any kind of a decision, and if I knew anything I would not be just an SHTA. They hate it. He laughed some and told me he would take care of it. It was a good thing he kept on top of it because it took almost another week before things finally got straightened out. Seems everyone was blaming the other and no one was actually fixing the issues. I guess that is just typical of the facility.

Things went on as if nothing had happened. I did send out a complaint through EEOC. I got a response from them asking me to clarify my complaints. I was also told that the facility was getting served within the week. It was funny that soon after that I had to go see Risk Management and give them a statement of what happened.

> I laughed at them and asked "What do you want a statement from me stating I did not know anything, and that nothing happened?"

> "We need a statement for the file. If that is your position on the alleged allegations then yes that is what they want."

A couple weeks later I got a letter stating that the allegations were disconfirmed.

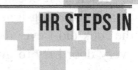

HR STEPS IN

HERE WE GO AGAIN ANOTHER canvas letter goes out, and of course soon after that a 70.1 transfer goes out over the facility email. Nothing too surprising here, after all the management is just trying to manipulate the list so they can get the person they want. I made sure my name is on the list and then I waited until the interview date. I am not energetic about the job posting or the chance of me getting selected. I am only putting in for it because of my pending law suit against the facility.

Even after all this time and things that has happened in the past concerning this job position openings, I still get a little on edge when ever new positions open up. I try to tell myself that it does not matter but I know deep down that it does. I guess the military instilled something in me that I never really forgot. You can hide for your past but your past will always be your past. None the less I try to stay focused and not to upset myself. My wife is right there on top of things to make sure I don't let it get the better of me. If anyone deserved a metal it would be her. How many spouses keep their soldier boy in line? Even though she sometimes gets on my nerves at times at how blunt she is when she lets me know how I am letting things get to me, I appreciate it. It makes me stop and think and ponder things. Sometimes I can handle things and deescalate on my own and sometimes I can't so I reach for the visteral. My wife says that I hide from the world and I drift away to my own world and become a zombie for a couple days when ever I grab the visteral. Of course there is some truth in this. I don't think I am trying to hide from the world so much as I am trying to not be in the world at that moment. For if I was in the world I would either have to except its unjust ways or fight for my sanity. Sometimes a little back stepping to gather your thoughts can make all the difference in the world to what happens tomorrow.

My anticipating interviews for promotion to SRSHTA always seem to bother me. Or at least stays on my mind all the time. I try and tell myself that I don't want the job so why get upset over it. I can not lie to myself so it doesn't work. It is not so much as getting a promotion as it is the being ignored and disappointed over and over again. What the fuck did I ever do to become such a black sheep here? Why does every door I try to go through for help always slam in my face? I get so tired of people telling me they support the military, yet do things to prove they don't? They don't want old soldiers around; they just want what the soldiers give them. Freedom, they like their freedom. They don't want to know what we soldiers do to keep their freedom. They don't want to know the truth. THEY CAN'T HANDLE THE TRUTH! Yet the funny thing is that I never asked for or expected to be treated special in any way. I just wanted to be treated fairly. I achieved a top score not on one test but two. I have great yearly reviews. I did not need to have an advantage of being a disabled combat veteran. That's the funny part. I did not need the help; I needed to be treated fairly. Hell it's been seven years that I have had a top score and I have been passed up over and over again yet I have no idea on how to better myself here. That is the most frustrating thing of all. They smile in my face and say how you doing yet they stab me in the back over and over again.

Now the supervisor's never gave any kind of reason for them not selecting me to advance to SRSHTA in the past, I believe that they didn't have a reason to tell me why I was not selected. Now with my frustration growing and my attempts to get any kind of an answer I did make my being disgruntle show. I can say that on one occasion that I did give them a good reason not to give me the job. Even I agree that it was not a smart move. I answered all their question at the interview as good and professional as anyone could have but my falling out came when they asked me if I had any questions. Sometimes it is better to just keep your mouth closed. I know this but on this day I knew which one of the SHTA that was going to be promoted because he was the best friend of the supervisor on the interview committee and I just had to say something. Of course once I opened my mouth and started talking it was hard to stop. I know I challenged his authority by confronting him on how he was going to make his choice and I attempted to get him to follow my lead and tell me why I would not be chosen. Of course he sat there all calm and cool and said the standard politically correct answer and that the most qualified person would be selected.

"Who determines who is the most qualified?" I asked

"It is not just based on test scores." He said. "Everything is taken into consideration. Your job performance, and your ability to get along with your peers, is just a couple of other areas that are taken into account."

"We all know that I have a chip on my shoulder over the past selections that you all have made. I am a retired MSG with 24 years of service where I served my country under fire and have a disability, and have higher test scores then the others and I have great yearly reviews. I have sought guidance on why I have not been selected in the past or how to better myself and all I have gotten is ignored! Your choice was already made before I even walked in this room and your holding an interview is just a joke."

With this said I excused myself and left. Of course this one time would be brought up as a reason why I have been overlooked for promotion time and time again. Of course they don't mention the numerous people promoted before this happened, or any of the issues that I have brought to their attention. My frustration over the way that I have or should I say have not been treated fairly has not been kept inside myself. I have tried over and over again for someone over me to do the right thing or at least tell me why I am such a black sheep. This time I wanted to make sure that I did everything right. Of course the fact that I knew I did not have a chance at the position took most of the pressure off me. After all what more could they do to me then what they have already done?

The interview started off different right from the get go. The first thing I noticed was the new AA lady. I personally did not know who she was but she used to work with my wife before and my wife spoke of her in a positive manner on how fair she was. Seems the last AA lady got promoted! Funny I did not think the last AA lady did anything to help anyone who filled a complaint yet she gets promoted. I wonder was it because she went along with management or shall we say got complaints to go away before they became issues. Or maybe it was that thing again. You know that thing that has me all confused as to what one was the actually thing that mattered the most, that she was a woman, black, fat, or just plain stupid. I wonder which one was the one that got her promoted. Maybe it was that old saying "you fuck up, you move up." Anyways I introduced myself to the new AA lady and shook her hand. I did not let on that my wife knew her, and that she felt that she would be fair, but it was a good sigh of relief for me that the new AA lady was there.

The next thing that stood out was the fact that all of the supervisors were present for the interview. This has never happened before. Maybe it is a meeting of the minds, maybe not. Nothing but show in my eyes, the rumors about who was going to be selected was already running through the building. I am sure they spoke to the people they wanted long ago just like always. Everyone knows that the interview process was just for show so they can say they gave everyone a fair chance. Fair chance is there such a thing, hell I would have a better chance of being selected if I played Russian roulette to get an offer. Hell then I bet it would be if the gun went off then I would get an offer. LOL such is life.

I sat down and notice a couple of papers in front of me. I picked them up as someone stated they showed what the pay raise would be. I put the papers down because I already knew all the answers it would say. You get a percentage of pay raise for every salary grade you advance. Pretty cut and dry for me, but I am sure others did not know. Then the supervisors stated that they had five standard questions that they were going to ask everyone. After the first question everyone started writing on their sheet and I asked if I needed a pen. Everyone got a good laugh, and the atmosphere of the interview just got better. I believe I calmly answered all of the questions calmly, directly, and with a little bit of humor all rolled up in one.

The interview was actually a nice pleasant meeting. Later I would get a couple of comments on how surprised they were and by how much I had changed. Funny I bet no one was more surprised at how the interview went then me, and as far as how much I had changed, I don't believe that my opinion on them or their promotion history has changed. If fact I would have to say that the only thing that has changed is how much I give a fuck about them or their promotion. I still bet that they won't select me. I guess time will tell the answer to that question. Or so I thought.

It was two days later when I got the word on the outcome of the interviews. Seems the chief and the supervisors were told by HR that their selection was not approved and that they were passing up people who were more qualified. You know how gossip goes, there is a little bit of truth and a little bit of added information mixed in. Funny thing is that it seemed that everyone of my co-workers that I spoke with were positive about this move by HR. You could hear the hope for something good out of them stepping in and not another good old boys club member who is just going to talk down to everyone and push people around just because he's a higher pay rate. You know that old saying that the boss is always right, well it is a shame that it is true because believe me the boss is not always right, or should I say the boss is not always right in my eyes.

Then I received this e-mail about a second round of interviews and if I was still interested in the job.

Good Morning,

You have been scheduled for a second Senior Security Hospital Treatment Assistant interview. Please respond to this e-mail confirming your interest. The interview will take place in the facility director's office. If you have any questions, please don't hesitate to contact me in HR.

Of course I replied to the e-mail that I was interested. I guess there was some truth to the rumor that the Chief and the supervisor's choice not being approved by their higher. The funny thing about being in charge is that you never really are totally in charge, there is always someone who oversee your actions or inactions, but if you are doing a good enough job you never really notice this fact. Seems management put up a big red flag to someone that their choices of SRSHTA have not been wise. What other reason could there be besides maybe HR wanting someone specific that was not chosen. If this was the case why not just say something to the Chief, instead of showing a power play.

A couple days later I get a call from one of our supervisors and he asks me if I received an e-mail about a second interview.

"Yes I have gotten an e-mail for a second interview."

"Was the e-mail to just you or was in a general e-mail?" He asked.

"I don't understand what you are asking?"

"Was the e-mail sent to just you or is there other addresses on it?"

"It was sent to just me."

"Have you heard of anyone else who has gotten an e-mail for a second interview?"

What the hell kind of a question is this for a supervisor to be asking me. I ponder this question before I answered him, even though I have heard of others why would he be asking me?

"No I have not heard of anyone."

"BULLSHIT! You took too long in answering that question. I know that you have heard something and you need to tell me."

"I got nothing to say. What do you want me to do start rumors?"

"That is why I am asking you Joe so I can put a end to the gossip and if it is a good rumor I will let it go."

"I got nothing to say to you. You are a grade 20 you should already know the answer to that question. Why are you calling me and demanding something that I can not give you?"

"I can't believe that after everything you won't tell me this. Come on now."

"I got nothing to say to you." I said.

What does he mean after everything? Not like we party together. How the hell do these people think they can shit on me and then talk to me as if they are my friends? Especially this certain supervisor who I have words with in the past. The harder he pushes the less he gets from me, but he too stupid to realize that yet. I mean he was almost threatening me on the phone because I would not answer him. The more he raised his voice the more I laughed inside. I guess the rumors of the supervisors and the chief not having any say in the promotions have some merit. I bet that is very embarrassing to them.

110

Of course the supervisor in question could not or would not let that be the end of our discussion. As they were making their rounds around the building he came over and sat by me. I knew he was there but I chose not to acknowledge him. What does he want to start an argument right here. I won't change my answer even if he is in front of me, does he not know that yet.

"Let me tell you what I have heard." He said.

What the fuck is this? Is he changing tactics on me after all this time? For him to just sit down and talk to me as if I am someone must be killing him. It sure is enjoyable for me, at least so far.

"I have heard that you and Xxxx, Xxxxx, and Xxxxxxxx have gotten interviews. Is that what you have heard?"

"I have not heard of anyone other then that." I said.

"OK then was that so hard?"

"It is not my place to tell you, you should be the one telling us."

"Well I have been off the last couple days and I am out of the loop. I do not understand why, but I am."

With this he got up and left. I never told him anything yet he believes that I had just confirmed what he told me. Funny he thinks he has outwitted me but it is I who has out witted him. What a fool he thinks he got his answer yet he got nothing. He just sat there and lied to me and we both knew he was lying because we both know of a fifth person who is getting a second interview. Now why would he not tell me about the fifth person? Secrets, secrets only smart people get to know that answer, and I am not in their smart person click.

A couple days later I went for my second interview which was held in the facility director's office. Present was just the director, HR personnel, and myself. The interview lasted half an hour and it was a very pleasant interview. The questions that these two asked were far more in debt then any of the other questions. Even though there was no right or wrong answers I am sure that they got a good impression of everyone they interviewed. Hopefully there will be some fairness out of this. The last thing that was asked is if I would take the job if offered. I told them I did not know that I would have to talk with my wife and that I never thought I had a chance before to even seriously think about it.

So I spoke with my boss (wife) and we came to the answer that I would take the job and we would see how it affected us with the kids. I don't think she wanted me to take the job, but she was not going to tell me no. I was not sure I wanted the job but was going to take it and try it out. Now all I had to do was to be offered the job. Now who could be a better choice then me, after all I have the top score, I am a disabled veteran, and I have been passed up for seven years without a reason. I must be a shoe in.

When I learned of the two who got promoted I was disappointed again to say the least. Actually it hit me harder then it had before. Maybe because I had decided to take the job and I had convinced myself that it would be offered to me. Then with all the fairness in the world the next day they congratulate one of the promoted ones as they move him to days and assign him over me. It is ok though I handled it like a champ, after all it was not his fault that he was promoted and I was not. What do you have to do to get promoted around here is beyond me because one of the ones who got promoted never even took the test and was not on the standing list at all. Fairness sure goes far in this facility.

This time I was not the only one who was upset over the selections, two people were very upset and stated they would never put for it again. Maybe they were asked before the canvas letters went out and were just waiting for it to be announced. I guess we will never know the true answer to that question. The other outcome was that the positive attitude that everyone got when HR stepped in was gone. Not only was it gone but it was worse then if they did not step in.

I could not get the bad taste out of my mouth so I wrote to the facility director. Not expecting anything just a chance to let my opinion know so I could get passed the big disappointment again.

Director:

I would just like to take a quick moment of your time to let you know how disappointed I was in the latest selection of SRSHTA here. I won't even attempt to ask why I was not chosen because I have grown tired of the non response that I have been receiving for the past seven years here. That is right I said seven years that I have had the top score on the civil service exam, and yet to be offered a position of SRSHTA. I have tried every avenue that I could think of to get both a reason of what I am doing wrong or how to improve myself so I would be able to someday reach that position. Still today I do not know the answer to that question, especially since all of my first line leaders have used me as their number one man. Even Xxxxxx Xxxxxxxxx when she was a supervisor on the 3-11 shift used me as her number one go to guy when ever she needed one. She even wrote it in my yearly review, and she went to bat for me to get promoted so long ago only be laughed at by the others. Her words not mine.

I am a disabled combat veteran who has dedicated 24 years of my life to the service of my country where I reached the rank of MSG / E-8. Maybe you don't understand how high that rank is but it is a much respected rank. I achieved that by starting out with the elite paratroopers and continued with the same drive that I learned there. I have always taken care of my men, and accomplished the mission as well. I am a certified small group leadership instructor in the service and have taught all NCOES levels.

I have had many deployments to many parts of the world and I chose to retire after my last combat tour of duty in Iraq. I will not even hit at me being some kind of hero, but I will say that I did what I had to do, and I made hard decisions that had to be made even during direct engagement from hostile forces. I have no regrets with any of the decision that I made though sometime I do wish maybe the outcome would have been better. I live with my ghost, as any one who has been in such a situation does.

I find it hard to understand how we teach our staff to see the signs of the mental patients here. Yet they fail to recognize a staff member who returns from combat and openly sought help. That is right I said I have openly sought help in the past here. If you look there is a policy on what to ask and what to do when someone returns from active duty. I do have a combat related disability that should have given me the priority in any civil service opportunity, and I also have even held the top score for the last seven years through two different tests, and still I am passed over! Every SRSHTA on nights except Xxxxxx has been promoted over me. Every SRSHTA on 3-11 has been promoted over me except Xxxxxxxxx. Two SRSHTA's on the day shift have been promoted over me. Not to mention those four or five persons that were promoted over me that no longer works here, and now by someone who has not even taken the test.

You asked me what goals I have in this facility and I say to you what goals would you think I would have at this time in this facility. I am more upset with myself then anyone else over this last round of promotions. I gave everything I had to the first interview and I know it went better then well. Still I did not expect to be offered a position but when HR and yourself stepped in and told the chief and the supervisor's that their selection was not good enough and you held the second interview I let my guard down because I felt I was finally going to get offered a SRSHTA position.

I could have lied to you and gave you every book answer there is to give. I was honest and truthful to you. I know that the disappointment that I feel in this facility must show through now and then. For this I make no excuses. I am who I am and I have my self respect. I would like to say that in the end all that happened was that I was passed up again, but the truth is that I did speak to my wife and I was going to take the position when it was offered. When I learned who was chosen I was very hurt and disappointed again. It tour at my insides, and my wife had to slap me back to reality again. I struggle to be that nobody that management wishes me to be. It goes against everything that the military has instilled in me to follow such poor leadership, and not change things. I have hung on to my sanity but this facility has lost so much more of a man then they will ever know. In the end we both have lost.

No response is expected or needed.

Now you know that any politician would have to answer this e-mail. After all if they did not then it could be said that it was ignored. Even though I stated no response is expected or needed I did look for it with anticipation. The response soon came.

Good Morning Dennis.

I genuinely appreciated your time during the interview process and as I stated during the second round of interviews we at this time had only two slots but many qualified candidates. I expect that we will have additional Senior SHTA appointments to make in the near future. Please continue to maintain your interest and commitment.

Thank you,

What a nice politically correct answer which said just about nothing. "Maintain my interest really!" That's what I am going to do, just what she said maintain my interest. I am going to maintain my interest in my law suit and not in the idea of ever being promoted or treated fairly in this facility.

18

LEADING HEALTH CARE IN THE 21ST CENTURY
MENTAL HEALTH RESOURCES AVAILABLE FOR VETERANS

THE CONFLICT IN AFGHANISTAN (OPERATION Enduring Freedom) and the War in Iraq (Operation Iraqi Freedom) are the most sustained combat operations the United States has been involved in since the Vietnam War. Our experience in working with the men and women who have been exposed to combat has shown that they are more at risk of developing Post Traumatic Stress Disorder (PTSD), Traumatic Brain Injury (TBI) and other mental health problems.

The Department of Veterans Affairs (VA), New York State Office of Mental Health (NYSOMH) and New York State Division of Veterans Affairs (NYSDVA) have collaborated to identify the broad range of mental health services that are available throughout New York State for veterans. This is designed to raise awareness about mental health issues related to combat and to identify resources that are available to veterans including women, active duty soldiers, National Guard troops and reservists.

Veterans returning from combat may have difficulty in identifying or discussing the problems they are experiencing (e.g., substance abuse, domestic violence, poor anger control, etc.). These concerns may be directly related to their military service. They may also be rooted in combat-related PTSD (Post Traumatic Stress Disorder) and TBI (injury to the brain caused by a significant force). Any of the problems mentioned above can negatively impact a veteran's ability to function socially, occupationally or educationally.

One of the problems veterans faced while overseas is that they would often go right back to duty after being involved in an explosion without awareness that an injury occurred and therefore not be aware that they may have TBI. Veterans with PTSD may think they have no problems related to the combat they experienced because the symptoms do not often present until the veteran returns home. That is why it is so important to ask about veteran status and to refer veterans to the following agencies.

115

General Military Service History

- Tell me about your military experience.
- When and where do you/did you serve?
- What do you/did you do while in the service?
- How has it affected you?

If your patient answers "**yes**" to any
of the following questions, ask,
"**Can you tell me more about that?**"

- Were you a prisoner of war?
- Did you see combat, enemy fire, or casualties?
- Were you wounded or hospitalized?
- Did you ever become ill while you were in the service?

Issues of Concern

It is recommended that all veterans be asked the following questions.

Post Traumatic Stress Disorder PTSD

In your life, have you ever had an experience so frightening, horrible, or upsetting that, in the past month you . . .

- Have had nightmares about it or thought about it when you did not want to?
- Tried hard not to think about it or went out of your way to avoid situations that reminded you of it?
- Were constantly on guard, watchful, or easily startled?
- Felt numb or detached from others, activities, or your surroundings?

VA Health Care Services

VA provides every active-duty soldier, reservist or National Guard combat veteran two years of free health care beginning on the date of discharge for all illnesses and injuries, unless clearly unrelated to military service.

The Veterans Health Administration (VHA) provides a number of health care services including:

- Primary care, inpatient, nursing home, and community-based residential care
- Dental, pharmacy, mental health, and prosthetic services

- Medical evaluation for military service exposure to environmental hazards
- Readjustment and vocational rehabilitation counseling
- Alcohol and drug dependency treatment
- Post traumatic stress and sexual trauma counseling
- Specialized health care for women veterans
- Health and rehabilitation programs for homeless veterans
- Domiciliary

Veteran Centers

Veteran Centers serve veterans and their families by providing professional readjustment counseling services to support post-war adjustment in the community. The Centers focus on counseling for military traumas, employment and family problems. Individual and group counseling is available for veterans and their families. Veteran Centers also provide referral services for VA benefits and medical services, and act as a liaison with community agencies.

New York State Resources

New York State has an extensive public mental health system that serves more than 500,000 individuals each year. The Office of Mental Health (OMH) operates psychiatric centers across the State, and also regulates, certifies and oversees more than 2,500 programs that are operated by local governments and nonprofit agencies. These programs include various inpatient and outpatient programs, emergency, community support, residential and family care programs. Veterans and their family members may access these programs through their local mental health system. The OMH Web site includes a tool that will help you determine the mental health programs available in your county. To access mental health services in your area contact your local County Department of Mental Health.

New York State Division of Veterans Affairs

The New York State Division of Veterans' Affairs was created to assist veterans, members of the armed forces, their families, and their dependents in securing benefits earned through military service. For more than half a century, the Division has been a strong advocate for veterans and veteran issues at the local, state, and national level. Web site: www.veterans.ny.gov

19

POST TRAUMATIC STRESS DISORDER

Post-traumatic stress disorder (PTSD);

- A mental health condition that is triggered by a terrifying event. Symptoms may include flashbacks, nightmares and severe anxiety, as well as uncontrollable thoughts about the event.
- Many people who go through traumatic events that threaten your safety or make you feel helpless have difficulty adjusting and coping for a while. With time and taking care of you, such traumatic reactions usually get better. In some cases the symptoms get worse or last for months or even years. Sometimes they may completely shake up your life.
- Getting treatment as soon as possible after PTSD symptoms develop may prevent long-term PTSD.
- Most people associate PTSD with battle-scarred soldiers.
- Military combat is the most common cause.
- Can affect those who personally experience the event, those who witness it, and those who pick up the pieces afterwards, including emergency workers and law enforcement officers.
- It can occur in the friends or family members of those who went through the actual trauma.
- It develops differently from person to person.
- Symptoms most commonly develop in the hours or days following the event, it can sometimes take weeks, months, or even years before they appear.

Traumatic events that can lead to PTSD:

- War
- Natural disasters
- Car or plane crashes
- Terrorist attacks
- Sudden death of a loved one
- Rape
- Kidnapping
- Assault

- Sexual or physical abuse
- Childhood neglect

The traumatic events that lead to post-traumatic stress disorder are usually so overwhelming and frightening that they would upset anyone. Almost everyone following a traumatic event will experiences at least some of the symptoms of PTSD. When your sense of safety and trust are shattered, it's normal to feel crazy, disconnected, or numb. It's very common to have bad dreams, feel fearful, and find it difficult to stop thinking about what happened. These are normal reactions to abnormal events. For most people, however, these symptoms are short-lived. They may last for several days or even weeks, but they gradually lift. But if you have post-traumatic stress disorder (PTSD), the symptoms don't decrease. You don't feel a little better each day. In fact, you may start to feel worse.

After a traumatic experience, the mind and the body are in shock. As you make sense of what has happened and process your emotions, you come out of it. With PTSD you remain in psychological shock. Your memory of what happened and your feelings about it are disconnected. In order to move on, it is important to face and feel your memories and emotions. The symptoms of PTSD can arise suddenly, gradually, or come and go over time. Sometimes symptoms appear seemingly out of the blue. At other times, they are triggered by something that reminds you of the original traumatic event, such as a noise, an image, certain words, or a smell.

While everyone experiences PTSD differently, there are three main types of symptoms:
1. Re-experiencing the traumatic event.
2. Avoiding reminders and numbing of the trauma.
3. Increased anxiety and emotional arousal.

Re-experiencing the traumatic event:
- Intrusive, upsetting memories of the event.
- Flashbacks (acting or feeling like the event is happening again).
- Nightmares (either of the event or of other frightening things).
- Feelings of intense distress when reminded of the trauma.
- Intense physical reactions to reminders of the event (e.g. pounding heart, rapid breathing, nausea, muscle tension, sweating).

Avoiding reminders and numbing of the trauma:
- Avoiding activities, places, thoughts, or feelings that remind you of the trauma.
- Inability to remember important aspects of the trauma.
- Loss of interest in activities and life in general.
- Feeling detached from others and emotionally numb.
- Sense of a limited future (you don't expect to live a normal life span, get married, have a career).

Increased anxiety and emotional arousal:
- Difficulty falling or staying asleep.
- Irritability or outbursts of anger.
- Difficulty concentrating.
- Hyper vigilance (on constant "red alert").
- Feeling jumpy and easily startled.

Other common symptoms of PTSD:
- Anger and irritability
- Guilt, shame, or self-blame
- Substance abuse
- Feelings of mistrust and betrayal
- Depression and hopelessness
- Suicidal thoughts and feelings
- Feeling alienated and alone
- Physical aches and pains

Just like the alcoholic who refuses to admit that they have a problem. The thinking that they can stop anytime they want, and that their drinking does not affect them or their environment. So does the person with PTSD. Or should I say so did I refuse to admit that I was not in control of myself. Even though I knew it inside, I did not, could not admit it. I knew that some of my feelings and actions were a little eccentric. I still refused to accept them as being out of control or of even that I have changed because of them. After all I am me. At least I think I am me.

NIGHTMARES

JUST WHEN THE NIGHTMARES STARTED is hard to narrow down. With all the working I was doing I never noticed that I was not sleeping. I just kept getting up and going in to work and then doing it all over again. I believe that when I finally did catch up to the bills and I stopped working so much and tried to take a breath is when things started to be noticed by me. I could not hide from myself anymore that I was having some issues. Knowing I was having issues with sleeping and nightmares was the most noticeable sign to me. It was kind of hard to say that I did not have a nightmare when I awoke full of sweat and heart beating a mile a minute. Of course the occasional bloody nose from the person next to me also helps some.

The nightmares became so bad that I was afraid to sleep. Afraid of what might be waiting for me. I was afraid of the feelings that I felt when I quickly woke up screaming or to the screams, and cries of someone else. Sometimes they seem to linger on for what seemed like an eternity, but only ten minutes or so in reality. It was hard to focus on what was real and what was not real. Was I dreaming that I was home or was I dreaming that I was in harm's way? Even when my mind started to clear the damage was done. Now I felt, and even believed that I was back to that god forsaken place. How does one come down from that rush? I had no way to calm down so I would just lay in bed afraid to fall asleep again or just shaking inside of me staring at nothing at all.

Times like that were made easier by some good old fashion illegal drugs. Snorting, and smoking made things easier to handle. Easier to cope with just lying there waiting for something, anything to happen. Better yet was drinking, smoking, and snorting before going to bed. The high was nice; it cleared my mind of everything except the solitude of being outside of me. In like a dream like state. I was just floating away, higher and higher. I was watching the game, of life from the side lines.

I remember one day I was at my mother's house which was by a hospital, and a medical helicopter flew in right over the house. I jumped off of the couch and said to my wife that "I felt like running in the back room and cowering in the corner". Then I just laughed it off. What a fool I was to be frightened by such a simple thing. My wife told me later that she had slept down some in the bed that night. It was a good choice on her part because in the night I had a nightmare and I swung as hard as I could and punch the headboard. The noise alone woke her, but the pain woke me. I felt as if my wrist was broken. I was scared. I did not know what to do. What could one do?

My answer was a simple one to do in my mind. I would just ignore things that are military like. Don't watch any war movies. Don't talk about anyone or anything that you have seen or done in the military. I grew my hair long, long past my shoulder blades. I colored it all kind of weird colors. First I colored it red then purple, blue, and even green. Anything I could do to not make me feel like I was ever a soldier I did. People always had smart remarks but I did not care. I was lost in my own hell and if coloring my hair made me feel even a little better than I was going to do it.

People would ask me if I was ever in the service and I would lie. I would say no. I would make up all kind of lies. Of course I sometimes got caught off guard. That really hurt. Not expecting it was the worse. It threw me back in time right at that spot and then all my memories that I tried to hide from would come flowing through my brain. They would crash into each other. All of them wanting to be seen, all of them wanting me to remember. It was like I was longing to be there, longing to get a hold of the things that I fought to forget.

The worse time was at work. A new nurse was talking about a young guy who worked at a hospital emergency room with her and how he died. He died in that hospital where he works. He died of a sickness. He was struck down early in his life. The nurse spoke of him and how his wife was at his side and how sad it was. Then she spoke his name. I stopped dead in my tracks and asked her what she was talking about, as I was not in the conversation just in the area of her conversation with another. He was a good friend of mine. He was our medical platoon sergeant in Iraq. He was our BN medical platoon sergeant at my National Guard unit. We have had some good times both while in uniform and out of uniform. Even now I can think of some of our conversations or our trip to Niagara Falls with the British soldiers. At our shoot fest before the British soldiers went home. The fun we had on our trip to Washington D.C. I don't think I ever had a bad word about him; he was always there to help anyone. I was devastated, even mad at myself. Why did I not keep in touch with my old unit? I was honored to have served with him, and to have spent those extra times together. To come home from war and then die was just a big tragedy. Now all of those memories kept flowing in my mind. To be replaced by the sight of his wife at his bed side as he passed away.

I did call my BN Operations Sergeant Major. He told me he knew that he died and that he was at his funeral. I felt so bad that I had missed it. How many others have passed or gone back that I don't know about? I spoke with him about how I felt about finding out like I did and that maybe I was wrong to just forget about everyone and everything. We spoke some about what was going on with both of us. He asked me how I was doing and he suggested that I should call the Rome VA, and that they had a good therapist there who knew how to handle PTSD with soldiers. I got the number and told him I would call, but like everything else it went out of my mind, and I did not do it.

Yes the nightmares are the worse. There is no hiding from them. You try not to sleep. You try to just take cat naps because they don't seem to come then. They are always on your mind. The nightmares are always lurking just a stone throw away. Sooner or later you know your body is going to crash and fall into a deep sleep with exhaustion. Until then you try not to think but you can't. You can't get any relief from yourself. What can one do?

SEEING THINGS

THIS IS A TOUGH ONE. How many times does someone think they might have seen something but when they take an extra look it is not there? How many times I questioned myself or just turned my head and laughed at myself. Maybe it was just my imagination running wild on me. Still the uneasiness always stayed with me. I could try and fool myself but I was the fool.

I remember when I moved into a new apartment down by the beach. Behind the house was nothing but woods and a swamp. One day in the kitchen I caught a glimpse of a figure all dressed in white. My first thought was that it was an anti-coalition force outside. I stopped. My heart was beating and I could not believe what I was seeing. I kept my eyes on it as long as I could. When the figure went behind a tree I moved so I would be able to watch where they were going. The feeling that I was being spied on ran through me. Maybe they were trying to sneak up on me? I spent ten minutes looking for where they went. I knew they were not there yet my brain told me they were.

The tug-a-war started, would it be my brain or my mind. My mind was telling me to get down! Get out! Run, grab the kids and just go somewhere else where we would be safe. Pick up the phone call 911. I am being attacked. They are surrounding me. HELP! I need help. I need fire power. Someone come and clear the woods for me. My brain on the other hand was telling me that it was unrealistic that someone was there. Someone could not disappear that fast. If someone was there you would still be able to see them. Sounds simple but believe me it is not a simple thing to convince oneself that oneself is wrong. That oneself did not see what one believes that they have seen.

If I believe that it happened is it not true? Is it not true at least to me? I believe that I am right. If I call someone will they take me away? Will they laugh at me? How can one argue with themselves over this? The voices inside of me are telling me two different things. What do you do?

Do you hear voices? What a question to ask someone. I mean is it that I am hearing voices or am I just talking to myself. Is it my conscious deciding what is right and what is wrong? Am I just trying to convince myself of something? Isn't it normal for someone to talk to themselves? Don't you see people doing it all the time? I would be asked this question later by my psychiatric. Do I hear voices? I told her I did not know and maybe she could tell me. She looked confused over this statement. I spoke maybe it was me talking to myself, my conscious. I asked her what she thought of what I said, and the answer I got was very surprising if not silly.

"Do the voices tell you to hurt yourself?"

"HELLO! I am here aren't I."

"Do you have a plan on how you would hurt yourself? Did you ever attempt it?"

I just laughed and said "if I was to attempt it I would not be here, because I own a 44."

"Now what does that mean?"

"Simple if I ever did try it I would not fail." She did not see the humor in this, and she would not answer the question that I wanted answered. "Am I hearing voices or is it normal to speak to oneself?"

Guess it is whatever one thinks. I know I talk to myself or I talk to someone inside of me, but I did not give my voices any names. I did recognize that there are three of them inside of me. So I got besides my own opinion three different voices telling me three different opinions on life. This I accepted and finally used it as a positive trait.

I would even joke about it to people that there was three people inside of me and there was no more room for anyone else.

To this day they are there. Don't know if they will ever leave me alone. At least this way I am never alone. I always have my friends with me. Right or wrong they always come along, and they are not shy about speaking their opinions of something to me. I even enjoy talking to them. I always have the last say and I have never let one of them decide anything. I am in control of me. At least for now I am in control.

MEMORY LOSS

"I don't remember that!"

HOW MANY TIMES DO YOU hear that excuse from someone about something that they were expected to get or do? The old trout look. Sound comical at times. Just think if it was really true. If one did not remember anything before today. Some might cherish that thought. That way they did not have to face up to anything that they did or said. On the other hand it of course could bring some surprises your way. Unfortunately I did not remember anything that happened before today. Maybe it was my brains way of not dealing. Of wiping the slate clean. I mean if you don't remember anything then how can you face it? Wish I knew how long I could not remember anything went on, but I can't remember!

This did not come to my attention until I was at my first therapist appointment. I must of really look silly to sit there and struggle with what I had done, or even ate the day before. To make matters even worse it was not just my memory of what had happened that was gone it was also my thoughts of tomorrow. There was no next week, or next month. I was living in the now. Now was all that I was, and at this point in my life all I was is a shell of a person all strung out on illegal drugs, and alcohol just stumbling through the days. Was a good thing I had someone to tell me what I was doing.

There was some good and some bad outcomes of not being able to remember anything; it's all depending on how you are looking at it. I did not miss my kids as much as I should of. It was not that I did not love them, because they will always be my little babies. Of course the wicked witch of the past (my wife) was far out of my mind. Did I want to forget or was my mind shutting down?

My memory loss did cause some problems here and there. Even my three friends (voices in my head) and I had some times arguing about what we did or where we put something. It was hard to know what reality was or what was just in my mind. Then the old question comes into play that if I believe it to be true then is it not true? Did it happen or not! This only started to bother me when I was starting to search for help. It's hard to change something if you don't remember it.

ANGER MANAGEMENT

Anger;

*   A feeling of great displeasure or hostility: wrath.

ANGER MANAGEMENT OR ANGER MISMANAGEMENT that is the question. Whether it's nobler to suffer the pain and anguish of the mind, or is it better to release your anger out on others, that is the question. \

Anger like any emotion is not bad if it comes in moderation. It helps us relieve some stress that otherwise would build up inside of us until we pop like a balloon. Normally we pretty much know why we are angry. There could be a lot of different reasons for different people depending on their values. What if you find yourself angry but you don't know why you are angry, and no matter what you do you are still angry? How does one deal with that? For me I tried to blame my anger at something or someone else. After all then I could justify my anger to myself.

Because of my anger management or mismanagement I would sometimes let the anger just fester in me till I did things to unwind sometimes without thinking about the consequences. I would do stupid things like kicking furniture out of my way at work or by being very rude to others. Sometimes I would feel like I was a bottle of nitro glycerin, just waiting for the wind to blow and break the glass so my energy would be unleashed on the world. Because of this I would always try to sit alone just me and my three voices, so I would not have to interact with anyone else. I would be angry for no reason at all and this seems too irate me even more then when I could peg my anger on something or someone else. I would think to myself that maybe I am just having one of those days, and since I did not remember yesterday I never knew I was having one of those days every day.

When I started to drink it seem to quench my anger right out of me. Then the drugs seem to numb them so I no longer was that time bomb ticking away. Now I became a bomb that was just waiting for something or someone to set the timer ticking. I was still dangerous but I was in a more controlled environment. Now that is funny if you think of it. Yet it is the truth. How many others are out there holding on by the seat of their pants or by the bottle they hold in their hand? How many never made or will never make it to the point of using drugs and alcohol to damper their anger? How many have taken, or will take that easy road out?

My anger was still there it was just under the ground some. Like that personnel land mine, I was just lying in wait. Would a trip wire get snapped to set me off or would someone or something step on me that was the only question to be asked at this time. Even though I would get mad or be mad at everything and anything, driving on the streets was by far the worst thing or time for me. What people would call road rage was in my mind Joe's rage.

ROAD RAGE

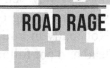

Rage:

- A violent anger.
- A fit of anger.
- A craze; fad. Fad.
- To be violently angry.
- To move or spread with violent force.

NOW THIS WAS SOMETHING THAT I noticed right from the start. This thing called road rage was there inside of me and it came spilling out time and time again. I never accepted it as road rage in the beginning; I would always blame my anger / rage at the other stupid drivers on the road. The drivers that are driving so slow in the fast lane and not getting over to let me go by them. To just not using their turn signals properly. It did not matter that I was the worse one out there not using my turn signals. I knew that I used them if I had to and that I did not turn slow so I should not be a bother to them. I am of course always right and every other driver out there is wrong or better yet stupid.

I even had my own set of rules that I followed that determined what kind of response they would get from me. I would always try to stay calm or at least I fought the urge to drive them off the road. Normally I would first tailgate them really close to get them to move. This tactic worked great in my truck but had a littler effect when I was driving a smaller vehicle. Next I would turn my lights on and maybe drive a little more left so they would see me wanting them to move over. If they still did not get out of my way I would start to flash my head lights at them. Finally I would start to blow my horn. Of course all this time I was screaming even if the only ones who could possibly hear me were in the vehicle with me. If I had to go this far to pass them I surely would be a bigger asshole than they were when I got in front of them. I would either slam on my brakes or go very slow and not let them pass me on either side. Following vehicles that I could not see around would never happen. I would always pass them, or if not stay way behind them. Of course the staying behind them always was very trying on my part. The passing was always the best option. Not really in a race to get anywhere but I was in a hurry to be in the lead and not follow anyone.

It seemed almost every time I was on the road I was getting very upset at something or someone. I hated driving even though I was driving lots and lots of miles every day. This did nothing to help me be calmer, if anything it made me more jumpy then I already was. I knew this but I had no idea of how to fix the problem or even that is was a problem. All those close calls I had to fighting or crashing were surely the fault of the other driver. After all if they were not on the road I would not have the issue with them.

You are most likely wondering why the road rage was so hard to handle. Over in Iraq there were no real traffic laws. No one to enforce the traffic laws that is. Whenever we were on the road we would not let any civilian vehicles in our convoy. There was ways of getting anyone who dared to mingle within our convoy from moving off the road. Sometimes it took just to show a gun or two. Sometimes it took a little more action like firing warning shots in front or to the sides of them. If this did not work we would shoot their Engines full of holes. Those person(s) who got shot or crash because of this was just an anti-coalition force in our eyes. After all those that don't help only hinder. Another way which is far my favorite way is to drive them off the road. That is what I said. We would drive them off the road. Non-aggressive at first but if they refused to move we would get a lot more aggressive to the point where our vehicles would touch and we would make them crash. Better them crashing then them being in our convoy to set off a bomb or shoot someone.

Of course the military were not the only ones over there driving as they wished. Iraq has one major highway going right up the Tigris River. It has four lanes. There are two lanes going each way with a small natural divider between them. When civilians would see a convoy on the road they would drive to the other side and go as fast as they could into oncoming traffic. Does this sound safe? Now take into account the number of different military convoys on a daily basis going each way and those civilian cars just zipping in and out of traffic. Just imagine the amount of accidents that happen on a daily basis. You can see why someone would be so on edge every time they got on the road. It is easier to take the soldier out of Iraq then it is to take the Iraq driving out of the soldier.

To this day I fight the road rage, and driving is one of the hardest things I accomplish without having any issues. I find that instead of turning the music up if I turn it down or just don't play any at all it seems to help keep me calmer. Medicine helps a lot and I always carry some vistaril in my vehicles. It is not a cure all, but a crutch that I rely on when nothing else works. Of course nothing helps when you got a vehicle full of teenagers trying to play their music and fighting over anything and everything. There is no help for these days. I do try not to be in such a hurry and I try to use my cruise control as much as possible. I even try to keep my speed even lower than the speed limits at times. It is hard and I am working on it. The wife and kids are always there to let me know when I am being stupid.

The biggest issue is after I get to the high state of emotions from driving how can I calm myself down to a point where I am really in control. Many of arguments have come between my wife and I because of how agitated I get. She thinks it is the kids. She fails to understand that it could be nothing but once the feeling comes I need help. I need some kind of help to unwind. Whether the help be medicine, quiet time, some alone time, or maybe just someone to talk to about it. After all I can't be the only one feeling this way now can I?

I know some of my triggers which my therapist says are the first part in solving or controlling the issue. I do try to stay in control. I do tell myself that it is stupid to be so angry over nothing. Sometimes it works and sometimes I have to use the Vistaril. Sometimes I cringe for a few hours or longer. I still want to drive the other cars off of the road. I still see the car flipping over and over down the incline at the side of the road. If life was so simple that all we had to do would be to just step on things that bother us. What a wonderful world it would be. At least until someone stepped on me.

Lonesome:

- Sad at feeling alone.
- Offering solitude; secluded.
- Sad at being alone.

BEING LONESOME OR HAVING LONESOMENESS is not what one might think that it is. I am not speaking about being all alone with no one else around. I am talking about connecting to someone, something, some reality to keep you grounded. Sounds pretty much like just fitting in. Fitting in is a real good description or should I say not fitting in is a good description of what I am trying to say.

Just imagine that you are in a group of your co-workers or friends. They are all laughing and joking over something. You are going through the motions here and there and making it look like you are with them. In reality your mind has your body in the distance looking over at them. You are not with them. You see your body with them but you are not in your body. You don't fit in anywhere and you are just hovering, waiting, even longing to get far, far away from them.

You don't feel anything when you feel lonesome like this. It is in itself a relief maybe even a new world. Maybe this is when I started to talk to those other voices inside my head. The voices and I were the only ones around. Sometimes even today I feel like I am apart from things that are going on around me. When I get in this state it is hard to grasp what is going on. Normally I would just go off in to my bedroom and watch some television or play on the computer. My wife will say something to me like go out there and do something with the kids you can't just hide in here when you can't handle things.

The hard part is sometimes I don't know what the thing is that I can't handle. Sometimes it is just the everyday stress that finds a way into my brain and starts to grow. Just like that ant hill in the back yard it grows and no one really knows, and when I do notice it sometimes it is too late. Sometimes I figure out or I know from the start why I am drifting but I am powerless to stop it.

It reminds me of when I went to Washington D.C back in 1982 for a ZZ Top concert. I was young and a paratrooper in the U. S. Army. I was not doing drugs regularly but I did take a puff here and a puff there. When the joint was passed around after the concert party I took a couple hits. My army buddy came over and yelled at me. He stated that I did not know what I was smoking. Oh is someone supposed to tell you when they lace a joint with LSD? I missed that class, and it was my first and only time that I ever had any LSD.

I still remember that day like it was yesterday. Wish I could say it was a nice trip, but I would be lying. I knew everything that I was doing because I was watching myself do it. It felt like I was above myself watching some other person doing it, yet I was the person doing it. I had no control of myself and I felt like a puppet. A puppet but no one held the strings that was making it do all those crazy and stupid stunts. Yet I could not stop myself from doing them. Does that sound crazy or stupid or what?

My lonesomeness was like I was not on this earth but I was a spirit watching what was going on around me. Sometimes my body would be in the present and sometimes even my body seemed to be off in the distance. My mind was a blank and I felt like nothingness. The problem with this is that the nothingness that I was did not want to be anything more than the nothingness that I was. I was content to be away in spirit from everyone else. The fact that I have a high pitch hearing loss from the army sure did compound this issue for me. It was easy to ignore, it was easy to pretend to be alone. Hell it was easy just to be alone. No matter who was around me, I was comfortable being alone in my mind. Alone I was most of the time.

Things changed as I was searching for a difference. When I finally accepted that I was hearing voices and those voices were someone or something other than me then I always had someone to talk to. I found I had someone to always be there with me. To this day they are with me. We all challenge each other to better ourselves. That one critter who wants to hurt me is kept at bay. He is going along in the background waiting for his chance. He is waiting for his chance to be the lead dog again. All I can do is to keep myself grounded and try to always improve my life and to find something to look forward to in the future. It is working so far.

20

SEEKING HELP

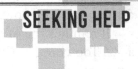

Help;

- To give assistance to (aid)
- To contribute; promote
- To give relief to ;help the needy
- To ease; relief medicines to help your cold
- To change for the better; improve
- To refrain from; couldn't help laughing
- To wait on; as in a store
- Aid or assist
- Relief; remedy
- One that helps
- A person employed to help

THE SEEKING OF HELP CAME for me when I was at my bitter end. I could stand no more and I either was going to kill myself or change myself. I could not have said it any simpler than that. I was at the cliff staring over. Or should I say I was staring at the barrel of my 44. It is hard to really say what goes through one's mind when they get to that point. Unless of course they just pull the trigger.

I know a couple times I thought of my x-employee John. John was a nice young guy. He was an avid bow hunter and John and I had many conversations on this subject. We both loved to bow hunt and we always got along since I first started working there. We were not working on the same ward anymore and he came to me and asked my opinion on what he should do. He was having a hard time at work, especially with his SRSHTA and a fellow SHTA who was assigned to his ward. He wanted to get reassigned because they kept taunting him over stupid stuff.

I asked him what he wanted his outcome to be if he moved to another ward, and I spoke of the what ifs. I mean things could be worse and sometimes it is better not to run away from your troubles but face them. Funny here I am giving advice that I surely don't follow myself.

Easier to give then to receive I guess. Anyway I did get him to stay on the ward and try to make the best of it.

Now I had gone through many changes in my hair and the way I presented myself, and one of the things that I did was I would tuck my pants inside my boots. Something all soldiers do, but I was doing it with my jeans. It did feel good. It made me feel strong, powerful, even on alert. John did ask me about how my pants were and I just laughed and joke back at him. I did tell him that whenever I tucked my pants into my boots that I was in an aggressive mood. It was true. It was like I was wearing my emotions on my sleeves, or should we say boots.

It was sometime later that I noticed John in the hallway before lineup and he had his pants tucked into his boots. It kind of made me chuckle as he was following my lead. I did ask him if he was ok, but I did not really pry into anything specific. We spoke about his ward and how things were going. He seemed content that he stayed there. I did say that I did not mind helping at that if he needed someone to talk too that I was there.

I was so lost in my own world that I did not notice the signs. The signs were all there. He was quieter. You could see there was something on his mind. His pants being tucked into his boots should have set off alarms in my head. He did not have a real smile on his face and you could hear in his voice that he was not energetic on this day. Like everyone else I just blew it off to John having a bad day.

A week later I got a phone call and someone told me that John was dead and that he had committed suicide. He had just bought a new hand gun and he used it to change his life. Does it really matter what you believe whether there is life after death or not? The cold hard fact was that he was gone and I felt like I had let him down. Maybe I should have gave him some more of my time, I should have listened more to him. I felt like maybe if I would have encouraged him to move off his ward and that things would look up for him. Instead I told him that things could be worse somewhere else and he should stay there.

John did leave a letter and he requested that no one from work be allowed to go to any of the services held for him. This only made me believe that his work environment and his co-workers were the ones who tipped the scale for him to move on. To this day I think of him often and wish I could have been there for him like he needed. I can also understand how he was thinking. I chose to fight. My kids were my ground that my feet wanted to step upon. I could not bear to hurt them anymore. I wanted to fix the issues that I created between them and me.

John is not forgotten. I still have John's pictures of the deer that he sent me long ago. I still have the frog email that when you look at it long enough it turns into an old wrinkly ass shot, and I look at it and laugh. It seems like such a simple and stupid thing to save but your choice made me angry. It made me angry at myself. My anger toward John was the beginning of the end of the hell I was living. My anger toward John made me want to matter to someone. I did not want someone else's anger to be on me for making the same decision. I knew I had to change. I had to change or I knew I would join John sooner or later.

John, I enjoyed your company and your stories and I wish you did not make that choice to go. I consider you my friend and I miss you, and think of you all the time. As my lighted arrow nock flies through the air I know you are always there.

JOHN

I enjoyed your company, and your stories
About your bow, and all its glory
You thought you were so smart
When your arrow hit it's mark
You always made me smile
Like that frog, which became that fat hog
And that funny deer that you cheered
I remember those tucked boots
I should of understood it then
And confronted you on your desire
Wish you did not chose to go
You will always be my friend
Rest in peace

EMPLOYEE ASSISTANCE PROGRAM

MY FIRST REAL STEP TOWARD changing my life for the better was when I went to talk to EAP. I was a little reserved when I spoke to him. He seemed to take the time to let me talk at my own pace. I tried to explain everything about coming home and dealing with my wife and the money and how I dove into work and how work was my happy place until I felt they were not treating me fairly. He asked me some specific to some of the things I said to him and he was the first to ask me if I thought about hurting myself. It was hard to say in the beginning. I still can see myself answering that question to him in a off handed manner. He picked right up on it though and kept me talking about it until I was openly telling him everything about my ideas and he wanted to know if I felt like it now. My answer was that I was trying to make the choice to make my life better and that I was choosing life over death.

He not only gave me the information about the Value Options program but he made me call right then and there. He wanted to make sure that I went through with making the call to Value Options and getting pre-certified so I could get some numbers on places to call. He had nothing to worry about. The hardest part was over. The hardest part was actually seeking out help from someone. Don't know how long I thought on this. Harder to get some action out of yourself then just your mind knowing what you should do. I guess it was still a teeter totter on which way I was going to go.

I left with a list of names and numbers to call. He told me to call him or any EAP representative if I needed to talk and if I could not get hold of anyone to call 911. I bet that would have been a funny call.

"Hello 911 what is your emergency?"

"Yes hello I don't know if this is an emergency, this is just little old Joe and I want to go."

"We are not a taxi service, if you don't have a real emergency and you just need a ride then call a cab"

"Oh. Sorry I did not mean to be a problem for you. I won't be a problem for anyone anymore so you do not have to worry about it."

"Excuse me. What did you mean by that? Where are you sir? Are you ok?"

Of course by this time the police car would already be dispatched to where ever I was, and if they made it in time to stop me, I most likely would have been admitted somewhere. No easier to just go and not call. After all I was not looking for attention, I was looking for me.

Any ways this did not happen. I did make a call to every number that I had and left messages on each machine. It was easy to choose which one to go to. I made the choice by the first one that called. It sounded simple enough, but I did not receive a call back for a couple days. Seems I was not the only one seeking help. When I did get the call I made an appointment to go and speak to a therapist. I do not know how a therapist would help me but I was willing to try and see which in itself is a giant step toward my discovery of who me is, and my issues.

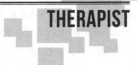
I WAS GIVEN ENOUGH NUMBERS and places to call so that I could change to another therapist if I felt uncomfortable with the one that I went to. I thought this was very funny in a way. After all if you go to someone to tell them all about how you are feeling and thinking are you not expose to be uncomfortable? I did call four different places and I only had one simple requirement for a therapist and that was for them to call me back. So I jumped on the first one who called me back and set up an appointment as soon as I could. Believe me time was not on my side.

Even though it turned out to not be a big place I still felt uncomfortable walking in. I was pleased to see no one in the waiting room. What I found there was that it was a small waiting room with signs all over to be quiet and respect others privacy. The room had a couple chairs on each wall and a rack of magazines. There were a couple of outreach fliers, and help lines. In the corner was a nice size water fountain with the water just a flowing out of a watermill. If this was not enough to make you comfortable there was some soothing noise / music being played. Some birds a chirping with the wind blowing softly. It was a very relaxing place to say the least. It was almost like heaven and I could have just sat there all day.

On the wall was a sign to fill out the in processing form and wait to be seen. I picked up a pen and a form and sat down to try and answer as many questions as I could truthfully. It was a little unsettling to answer the type of questions that were being asked of me. The form did not waste any time after the standard who are you and where do you live it got right down to what do you think are your issue and what symptoms do you have. The form had a list of symptoms and asked you to circle any of the ones that you have.

The therapist came out and took my form and then disappeared into another room. Maybe it was my answers because she was right back in a hurry and hurried me away to her room. She invited me to come in and get comfortable on a couch. Of course I had to ask her if she wanted me to lie down or not. She told me I could sit or lay down what ever made me more comfortable. Again with the comfort zone, I surely was not comfortable I was very uneasy and unsure that this would even do me any good. I don't think laying down would of helped. As a matter of fact I think if I did lie down I would have been even more uncomfortable.

Her room was a bit small, and a little congested with files and a fax / copier machine. She introduced herself to me and asked me how I was doing and if I really had all these symptoms. Of course she asked me that all important question. Do you feel like hurting yourself? She told me if I ever thought about hurting myself to call her and if I could not get through to call 911.

The next hour was filled with a bunch of questions about where I work, about my family, my military service, my childhood, any drugs that I was taking. The entire life of me all wrapped up in an hour long session surely would not work. She got the overall picture about my mind set. Maybe she even got a good idea on where to start, or maybe she was glad when the hour was over so she could think.

She wanted another appointment in a week and asked if I had any problems with trying different things. I told her I was going to give this 100% of my effort doing anything she suggested because I was at the end of my suffering and that if I did not change things for the good I would just end it and soon. There was no other choice that I had it was up or out and I was attempting to choose life over death. She had to believe me by the matter of fact way that I spoke of everything. I was not a human being at this time, I was just a shell that was empty and if it was not filled it would surely just blow away in the wind to never be seen again.

The next time I was there I realized that the place was set up so that the person who she was talking to in private could leave without the person in the waiting room seeing them. I now thought that instead of just a small place it was a nice cozy comfortable place that was strategically set up so ones privacy would be given to them. I was not worried about who saw me but I was a little bit curious about the type of people that came there. Were they all nuts? Could I tell they needed help if I saw them on the street? I never did see anyone leave. I did hear them. Like rats scurrying around after dark. Is that what I was to her a rat. Was I her rat that she could use to do tests on? Where is the maze that she will have me do? Am I even up to doing a maze?

Don't know but what I do know is even though I laughed at some of the things she made me do I was amazed at how I felt after leaving my appointments with her, and how I thought of them after. Hell I still smile and giggle some at how stupid I must have looked to her doing what she wanted me to do. Wonder what collage had taught her these things? Could have been an on line test. Surely Harvard would not teach such tactics.

One of the first things that I remember doing at the Therapist's office was to tell myself that I was somebody who was important and that I liked myself. Does this sound simple enough? Well of course it could not be that simple. She had me tap myself about every inch or so starting from the top of my head and working down to my chest. Each time I tapped myself I would repeat the phrase. Sounds stupid and I surely must have looked silly, but tap away I did. I chuckled at myself at how I must look. If only there was a mirror I could have really gotten a funny view of myself. Believe it or not I thought about this after I left and I did chuckle some more. I could not believe that something so silly would make me feel better. Guess all I needed was to tell myself I was someone to change things.

We were still on weekly visits and I was finding myself looking forward to them. She never told me to stop drinking or doing illegal drugs. She would ask me how things were going at what was new in my life and how I felt about this and that. It was good just to talk openly and not to worry about what I said. She made me think by the questions that she asked. I was starting to think. Thinking was something that I had hidden from before. Before I just followed the leader and lived for them. Now I was starting to see that I was not in control. Of course I knew this, but knowing and admitting are two different things. Now I was starting to admit that I know, but I was still along ways from taking total control of myself back again.

She did send me to a psychiatrist around this time to get me some medication as she could not prescribe any.

She asked me if I did not mind trying a new therapy that she had read about using colored lights. Again I thought she was nuts but I was willing to try it if she wanted me too. It was just a regular flashlight but she had different colored lenses to put in it. All I could think of was it was just like the military where you would change the different colored lights for signaling and OPSEC (operation security). I don't recall which color it was but she switched between her colors and I felt nothing until this one colored burned, no absorbed into my skin. I don't know how else to explain it. It was like the sun rays and it was transferring some of its energy right into me. I don't know maybe it's a known fact that a certain color will do this. Maybe she was just trying to make me believe that she was full of such knowledge that she could fix me. All I know is that it worked! Not only did I feel the energy but the simple fact that I did feel the difference with the different color light, and that made me so amazed that I laughed at how stupid it was. I still remember the moment, and I still laugh at the thought of myself. Guess we can chalk that new study up to a positive one for me.

We continued our secessions going from every week to every other week. Things must be looking up for she thinks we can go longer in between visits. Maybe she is getting too much of me? Maybe she needs a break from me? I know I need a break from me a lot of times. I am feeling better after talking with her. It is a great relief to me. She tries to push me a little farther each time we talk. She keeps trying to get me to stop using the alcohol and illegal drugs. I am not there yet. I still need the comfort that they have given me. At least now I am thinking about staying around a little longer.

My childhood is brought up and she thinks that maybe I should write each of my parents a letter about all the unsaid feelings that I have toward them. It did give me something to think about. She said I did not have to give it to them, that I could just keep it for myself and that just doing that would make me feel better. Just to write it down would help me accept things maybe even think more about them. Maybe that is the key she has been trying to get me to turn all this time, just to think about the things, and to get them out of that locked chest. Maybe I need to unlock my far past also. To ask myself why I am like I am. But am I not already talking to those others in my head? What possible good could come from writing to them?

Like I said before I was giving it 100% of my effort, so I thought I could do better then write a letter to my parents especially if I did not plan on giving it to them. They are divorced and they live 300 miles apart. They were married for sixteen years but it was a trouble marriage as far as I remember. I remember the drinking no the drunkenness that went on every day. The beatings that my mother took from my father that gave her black eyes, and bruises. I remember my mother seeking companionship from others and attempting suicide in the end. I should have known that she overdosed because we were learning about it in school. My big brother came to the rescue and called for help. My mother would say later in life that my father knew what she had done and that he had left her there. When she got out of the mental hospital she took four of her five kids with nothing but the clothes on our backs and moved away to another state. She tried to get help through the Salvation Army but they would only take her and two kids. My mother was not going to choose between her kids. Her brother came and got her and off we went.

Would have been a hard move for anyone going from a small urban city to a great big city, but if you take into account all we had or did not have and that we spent two long weeks at a drop in center before my mother could get any assistance and that I was so naive hell I never even seen a black person before and now I was in a school where the whites was the minatory.

First I called my mother since she was in another state and spoke to her on the phone. It was not as simple as that but you could see that we both were being honest to one another and telling our story from each others perspective. We both learned things that we did not know. Funny how two people can see the same thing and yet have two different opinions of what happened or why it happened. I know she was living her own nightmare. Her moving us away was her chance at life. I guess her attempt at death sparked her ability to make the move. Funny how sometimes you realize that what you are thinking or doing in your past was just silly, stupid or down right selfish.

Talking to my mother has brought us closer together. She has apologized many times for being a rotten mother and of the things that have or have not happened long ago. I tell her that she has nothing to apologize for. Choices were made by everyone according to what they believe. I don't hold any bad feelings toward my mother. As a matter of fact by talking to her has brought both of us closer. When memories from our past are brought up we don't hide. Sometimes we laugh and sometimes we cry but we are always by each other's side. Now isn't that what life is expose to be about.

My father on the other hand was different. I went to his house and found him with my cousin putting paneling up. I told him I wanted to talk and he said go ahead. I declined and said I wanted his complete attention. Him and I went to the kitchen and spoke. My father failed to acknowledge anything that happened in the past. Either he did not remember or he just did not want to face the truth with me. He talked as if our family was perfect until my mother took us kids and left. He said he never hit her and that he did not know what I was talking about. I was dumb founded, and at a lost for words as I sat there. After I left my father started bitching about me to my cousin. To this day there is that emptiness between us. Something I wish was not there but I can't allow him to not admit what I know to be the truth.

Today my father and I do get along. We fish, golf. Hunt, and play cards like any family. We have never mentioned anything about the past or of that conversation that we had. I guess something's are just better if they are kept unspoken.

Yes I can say that seeing this therapist did help me and that I would recommend anyone to see one if they are having troubles that do not seem to go away. It was a good start to my self control being given back to me. It is a lot of work though. Do not think that you do not have to put the effort into seeing a therapist, because you only get out what you put in. I went there at the end of my life, I knew I could not go on and I was ready and willing to try anything and everything that was suggested by her. Many people say it but I don't think they actually mean it. I lived it, I did it, I needed to change me and my life, and there were no short cuts. I was past the short cuts. I was on that thin wire wondering which way the wind would finally blow.

PSYCHIATRIST

AS MUCH AS TALKING TO the therapist was helping me it did nothing to stop the feelings or the nightmares from coming. Yes I was accepting that I needed some help and was seeking it so I did as I was asked to do and went to see a psychiatrist. Funny part was that when I sent up the appointment I had no idea that the doctor they were sending me to was one that worked at the facility that I worked at. It made it a little more awkward but none the less I was there and I went through with seeing him.

He asked me what was going on and again I explained it as simple as I could. Again with the standard question and answer period, it was getting easier in a way to talk about things anyway. He gave me a prescription and tons and tons of samples to use. I thanked him and away I went.

He put me on Wellbutrin which is an antidepressant. It made me calm on the outside, but I was still boiling on the inside. Kind of funny being so mad yet you don't show it anywhere. I think it was better then being high in some ways. When you are high things get all blurry. Here I knew everything that I was feeling and thinking yet I did not care. Of course that was good for some of my issues but not all of them.

Next he put me on lexapro which is also an antidepressant. This gave me the energy or the urge to do things. Both of these medications seem to be making a noticeable difference in my ability to control myself. The amounts had to be adjusted a little but together they seem to be helping.

I had to switch Psychiatrist because the one I was seeing started his own practice. My therapist gave me a number to one that she said some people have a hard time hearing what she is saying, but that she was a good one. I was a little concerned since I have a hearing loss but I called and set up an appointment anyway. It turned out that she was very easy for me to hear what she was saying, and that I was very comfortable with her, and she was nice to look at as well. Of course this bothered me every time she stood at the door to close it as I came in. I always said something to her that she did not have to stand there but she always did.

My meetings with her were always kind of short. She would ask me what was going on and how I was doing. She always asked about the illegal drugs and the drinking. She never told me to stop but did say that they worked against my psychiatric medications. She would listen to what I was saying and even took my opinion on adjusting my medication. Funny she goes to college to learn how to listen to me tell her how to adjust my own medications.

The Wellbutrin and the Lexapro did nothing to help with my sleeping so I asked and was given a prescription for Ambien, which is a sedative and is used for the short-term treatment of insomnia by helping you fall asleep. The Ambien had no effect, I was like those zombies at work, taking all kinds of medication to sleep yet they had little effect on me. So she took me off the Ambien and gave me a prescription for Rozerum, which is a sleep aid that is exposing to work with your body's internal clock to promote sleep. Of course the side effects are worsening of depression, suicidal thoughts and completed suicides, hallucinations, and nightmares. Maybe it is a good thing that Rozerum did not work to help me sleep. Someone at work told me they take an extra dose of Wellbutrin to help on those down times, so I tried it. It seemed to work but when I told my psychiatrist that I was taking extra Wellbutrin when ever I was agitated she was not happy. She said that it did not work that way and suggested that I go on something like Vistaril, which is used as a sedative to treat anxiety and tension and to treat allergic skin reactions. I laughed at this and made a joke that all I needed now was some Thorazine and I could have a cocktail like they give at work.

The Vistaril was nice. I did have her split the doze in half later. Sometimes it would knock me out and sometimes it had little effect. With the smaller doze I could control my reactions better. It was working. I always kept some with me at work, as I was driving, even at the golf course.

Things were looking better. I started to use the illegal drugs and the alcohol less and less. She seemed pleased with this, although I always asked her to take me off the drugs. It was something that I did once or twice in the beginning by myself. To stop taking them when I felt in control and then start again three days later when I was starting to get agitated again. It is the same thing that the patients at work do. They think they don't need the medication once it starts to work.

Even though I was doing better and I was using the illegal drugs and the alcohol less and less, and taking my prescribed meds like they were ordered, I still had a hard time sleeping. Worse yet was that when I finally got to sleep those dam nightmare were there waiting for me. I was still swinging out and hitting the person next to me. My psychiatrist told me there were no medications for the nightmares. I accepted this and thought I would have to go the rest of my life with having them.

She would always bring up the VA. She thought someone there should be more certified in dealing with the PTSD from the war. I was still in my denial from the service and I did not want anything to do with the VA at this time, besides things could not be better. I was getting my life back together and I was handling all the stress better. The worst part was the nightmares, and the big question is, was it worse for me for having those dreams and reliving those moments, or was it worse for the person I punched?

LAWYER

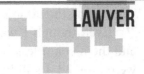

FINALLY I COULD NOT GO unanswered anymore and since I could not get any answers at work I sought guidance from a lawyer. She was not quick to accept my case though she explained to me how only people who fit into a federally established category can have a hostile work environment. Or should I say that you have to fit one of these categories to have a legal right to fight for any injustice that you feel has happened. How funny is that? Only minorities can be treated badly! Justice how funny? Guess that is why you hear that old saying that "justice is blind." Is it blind or is it just that it moves so slowly and cost so much that most people give up on the system before they get to any type of real justice.

She told me to think about it some more and make certain that I am sure about what I want to do, because things could get worse for me at work if I filed a complaint, and I told her that things could not get any worse and that I do not care what it cost. I was willing to pay it even if it meant spending money for a judge to tell me that I am unworthy of doing the job. The point of not getting an answer was worse then them passing me up.

She picked right up on my determination and gave me her opinion on the percentage of a chance of winning my case. told me that it would take $5,000.00 just to start the paper work. The $5,000.00 covered a non refundable retainer of $2,000.00, and $3,000.00 toward actual work to start. I went right out and borrowed from my state retirement. How funny is that? I borrowed from the state to sue the state. When I paid her the money she told me it could cost up to $10,000.00 if it went all the way to court. All I said was if she would of told me that I would of gave her the entire amount. Either way I did not care. After all it was just money. People throw money away everyday over nothing, and this was something to me. Well spent money, because I was fighting for me.

Speaking to the lawyer showed my ignorance toward the justice system and gave me a better way to handle things. I actually had to say to her to slow down and talk to me like I was stupid because I was getting confused when she started talking about AA (affirmative action) and EEOC (Equal Employment Opportunity Commission). She explained to me that AA has 180 days to make a determination, but you only have 180 to file a lawsuit, so if you wait for the AA to make a decision and think they will be your best avenue of approach, you might get left out in the cold. If you don't file a complaint through the EEOC with-in 180 days of the incident the time limit will be over you wont be able to obtain a Right to Sue letter.

I followed my lawyer's guidance and I was willing to pay any price or wait as long as it took to get my self respect back. As of the time I was writing this in the year 2012 my case is still pending. Like I said the wheels of justice turn slow, but they are turning, and I am fully prepared to keep them moving no matter what the cost or how long it takes.

AFFIRMATIVE ACTION

Affirmative Action:

- A policy seeking to re-dress past discrimination by ensuring equal opportunity.

  - **Equal:**
    1. Of the same measure, quantity, or value as another.
    2. Possessing the same privileges or rights <equal before the law>.
    3. Having the necessary strength or ability <equal to the task>.
    4. One equal to another.

  - **Opportunity:**
    1. A favorable combination of circumstances.
    2. A chance for advancement <a job opportunity>.
    3. Break, change, occasion, or opening.

  - **Re-dress:**
    1. To rectify: remedy.
    2. To make amends for or to.
    3. Satisfaction for wrong done.
    4. Correction.

  - **Policy:**
    1. A written insurance contract.
    2. A principle or course of action chosen to guide decision making.
    3. Prudent management.

THIS ATTEMPT TO BREAK DOWN Affirmative Action into smaller aspects of it is so one might see or try to see the real meaning of what it was set out to be. In reality we all know that this is never as easy as that. How could there be with the history of our country or the history of mankind? There always is someone who uses the system to give them the better edge. I mean if things were equal across the board then anyone could have a hostile work place. In our society only someone who fits a federal category of minority can have a chance of even addressing something that they feels is unjust. How lame does that really sound? Even if all men are created equal they surely are not treated equal and I don't believe they ever will be.

The reality of it is that there is no justice because there is always a policy written that even if it hopes to right the wrong fails to do the one thing that is needed. In my eyes it seems so simple. Why can't we all just say that there is no more minorities? Why can't we just do a mulligan and have a fresh start? Could that be the magical answer that will never be because some minority will have to give up their edge?

I don't mean to take away from the wrong doings that have been done in the past. The magnetite of what has transpired with the slaves, the Jews, the Indians. When or how can we ever be equal if there is not one set standard? How simple could that ever be? How much hatred is in the world just because there is policies set to right the wrong? In doing so are they not doing more wrong?

I use to think that I was not prejudice, but in reality I know that I am one of if not the most prejudice person on this earth, at least in my mind. I don't mean that I think any one culture or race is the master race. After all are we not the melting pot country? Are we not all created equal? So why can't we all be treated equal? When someone says that they are African American to me I usually tell them to go back to their home land, maybe even offer to pay for the boat. Yes I am a bigot. For I believe in the Constitution of the United States and that all men are created equal, and anything other then having all mankind treated equally is an injustice to me.

So it must come as no surprise to anyone that I don't agree with Affirmative Action, but it is there so I did attempt to use it to see if there is some kind of justice for someone who is not treated fairly as others. Of course when you fill out the form you see that the policy is only there for those who fit the federal category of a minority. I am a Caucasian American male, so I don't fit any of those categories or so management must have thought. I am a veteran and I did file the complaint under that category, but of course all of the policies are set up for Vietnam Area veterans and nothing is written for any of the current actions that have taken place since then. So again someone must have thought there was no standard that I could complain about through the Affirmative Action policy. Through my searching of an answer I learned that even if someone is perceived to have a disability in the eyes of the law they have a disability. Finally I have a leg to stand on; even if no one believes it hell I did not believe it because in the beginning I refused to admit that I had a problem of PTSD.

Now if one was to look at the definition of AA they would see that the policy was written to address past discrimination to ensure that everyone was treated on the same principles. Of course this only goes for minorities, another catch 22 in these complicated times. I knew that I was treated unfairly and I wanted someone to stand by my side. I did not think that I was asking too much.

So I made out a packet of all my yearly reviews, my test scores, my e-mails and conversations that I have had in the past seeking guidance and asking why I have never been approached on a promotion. Of course the AA lady took her entire 180 days that she has to review the complaint. Maybe management thought I was stupid and would not cover all avenues, but I did by writing to EEOC at the same time that I filed the AA complaint. One would think that with all my e-mails and conversations that I was not going to let it go until I got an answer.

Of course she took her time in giving any kind of a response; it seemed that she was more focused on the future of my job performance and very little of what I was actually complaining about. Her answer to me was that I had filed a law suit and that I should let it go and think about today and not yesterday. Not yesterday, hell it was still today the shit was still going on. How can AA personnel say to someone to forget about the past and your feelings of being discriminated / humiliated and find a way to be happy and satisfied with my job and with my upper management personnel? I would have many conversations with the AA lady both in person and in writings.

I remember on one occasion when I went to see her that really set the tone for all of her actions in dealing with me. The state had sent out a canvas letter for a SRSHTA in the facility. When the facility got the list of interested people on it they saw that there was three 90's on the list that were in the building and they did not want any of them. So in order to manipulate the list to get who they wanted the facility requested two different SRSHTA positions that had weird hours and weird days. So the state sent out two more canvas letters, hoping that one of the lists will not have the three 90's on it. That way they could hire off of either list. Of course they were not fooling anyone and the three of us got together and made sure that all three of us sent the canvas letters back saying we were interested in the job. This had two effects. One the SRSHTA's in the building put in a grievance on the fact that the facility was offering SRSHTA job with different pass days and different hours without going by seniority. Two the facility then sent out a memo for a 70.1 transfer. WTF how can they do this?

So I went to the AA lady and explained what was going on as an example of how the facility was not treating people fairly. Now remember that the AA policy was established in order to re-dress past discrimination by ensuring equal opportunity for all. So she tells me with a straight of face as possible that they have the right to do that under Civil Service law. I was confused and I asked how that could be right.

"How do you think someone like me got a job like this." She said.

I just looked at her; it must have been a trout look on my face. I could not speak because I was surprised by her answer. After all she is the AA for the facility and now she is telling me it is ok to manipulate the list and not have equal opportunity for everyone. Running through my mind was what was she talking about? Was it the fact that she was fat, black, a woman, or just plain stupid that got her the job? How can I ever get a fair review of what has transpired to me if this is how she thinks?

The policy states that the AA personnel have 180 to make a determination on a complaint. My 180 days came and went and I had to repeatedly request her answer or her findings.

On 4-17-2011 I wrote to AA:

AA

I was wondering about the complaint that I made and when I would receive notice of the outcome of the complaint.

I got a reply on 4-21-2011:

Joe,

A quick note to let you know that I am out on the road, but will be in touch when I return to the facility.

I wrote back to AA on 5-8-2011:

AA:

   I know u a busy person. Just wondering if u had an idea when u would return to the facility?

I got a reply from AA on 5-9-2011:

Hi Dennis,

   I am here for part of this week, so I will prepare your determination letter and get it in the mail. Your patience has been greatly appreciated. Let me know if you want to stop by and talk.

5-9-11 I wrote back to AA:

AA:

   I would prefer to see you and discuss your determination. I hope this does not cause any problems for you.

She set a date and had me come to her office to tell me that she found no grounds of discrimination. I was shocked a little, I mean I expected this answer but I also down deep wished for some kind of justice. I did not understand why she did not have her findings written down and she stated to me that she thought because I agreed to see her to discuss her findings that she did not have to put it in writing. WRONG! How could anyone think like this especially with the amount of time and effort that I had put into having everything documented. Maybe she did not want to commit herself to an answer in writing but I was going to get it in writing. She then told me she would have to have the facility director sign it and then she would send me a copy. Yea whatever!

A couple weeks go by and I do not receive the official written answer so I call her and she tells me that since I saw her in her office to discuss the outcome she did not think I wanted it in writing. No I said you said you were going to get it signed by the facility director and then send me a copy. She said she did not say that but that she would get it signed and then send a copy to me.

FORM xxx AND (xxx)(XX-XX) State of New York
To be completed by Affirmative Action Officer Office of Xxxxxx xxxxxx

DISCRIMINATION COMPLAINT DETERMINATION	
To: Mr. Williams	**Date:** 07/06/2xxx
RE: Claim No: 252-2010-xxxxx	**Based on:** Disability (regarded as having) Military Status

We have conducted a thorough investigation in your claim of discrimination. Based on Our findings, we have made the following decision:

There was insufficient evidence to substantiate your claim.

RECOMMENDATION:

Refresher training for security Department staff.

Please call TxNxxxxxx Wxxxxxxxxx if you need further clarification of this determination.

Sincerely, Mxxxxx Bxxxx
(Agency / Facility Head)

FINAL RECOMMENDATION:
DISMISSAL __X__ **REMEDIAL ACTION**_____ **COMPLAINT WITHDRAWN**_____

DATE OF FOLLOW-UP: Completed **SIGNATURE:** xxxxxxxxxxxxxx	**DATE:** 07/06/2xxx

THIS DOCUMENT IS PART OF AN INVESTIGATION AS SUCH, IT CONTAINS CONFIDENTIAL INFORMATION AND IS MEANT ONLY FOR THE USE OF THE DESIGNATED RECIPIENT. PLEASE DO NOT DISSEMINATE THIS DOCUMENT OR ITS CONTENTS.

To say that the findings were an insult to me is being mild. I could not believe what I was seeing. Just one sentence, "There was insufficient evidence to substantiate your claim.", and then she recommends "Refresher training for security Department staff." What a fucking joke. I see that there is fairness here. She could have at least addressed a couple of my concerns in detail. Surely she does not expect me to accept this answer as anything more then a piece of shit paper to wipe my ass with.

I felt I had no choice but to appeal her decision to Albany. Albany AA called me and talked to me on the phone stating that the file has been reviewed and that they agree with the decision that was handed down. Of course I had to get my side of the story explained in more details. Surely someone must be able to see that I am grasping for some kind of justice no matter how faint it might be.

I brought details about who they hired and how they had hired them. The number of people that were hired over me and the fact that for years I have been asking why and how to better myself in the facility and that I have not gotten any response at all. Albany said she would look into and that she would get a list of everyone who was promoted since I was reachable and that she would meet with me then to discuss it more. I agreed and waited for her to get back to me.

In the time that I was waiting for a response from Albany AA I sought assistance from my facility AA in dealing with what I thought was an unfairness to me over an locker issue that was discussed in Chapter 16-11. Maybe the AA lady's opinion was that she was trying to foster better communication between management and myself (which is something that I have tried to do with management since the beginning), I never felt as if she ever truly wanted to fight for the injustice that I felt had happened in the past. Is that not her job to deal with the injustice? Maybe she would be a better Human Resources personnel then she is an AA personnel?

Let's give her the benefit of the doubt again. The next time I sought her assistance is when the SRSHTA tries to get other SHTAs to file false complaints against me in retaliation for not following his orders to move my locker. Surely this fits into her realm, after all AA is exposing to deal with discrimination based on:

- RACE
- COLOR
- NATIONAL ORIGIN
- CREED

- AGE
- SEX
- MARITAL STATUS
- RELIGION
- RETALIATION
- DISABILITY
- ARREST RECORD
- CRIMINAL RECORD
- SEXUAL ORIENTATION
- VIETNAM ERA VET. STATUS

For her to tell me that it does not fit into her area of expertise and to have me send it through Human Resources was just another example of her not doing her assigned job as an AA representative. Was this not an obvious case of retaliation? My disbelief and my feelings of aloneness just kept growing the more and more I sought justice or fairness from some other state organization.

It took a couple of months but finally the lady from Albany came to my facility and met with the AA lady and myself. I was looking for a little down to earth answer about what has gone on and why I was given the answer of unfounded to my complaint of discrimination. What I got was someone who told stories that attempted to show me the meaning of life.

One story was about grandma's house and that to get there you had to take the right road, and if you took another road you might not ever make it there. I think what she meant was that I had to go along to get along. I told her that I did not have to take the same road as everyone else and that if I had to take the same road maybe I did not want to get to grandma's house.

Then she started talking about two rams high on the mountain top. Two rams butting heads to see which one was the more dominant. One ram has to step down or they will just keep butting heads until one or both of them dies.

"I must be a ram then because I refuse to give up to any of the wrong doings that have happened to me without an answer from someone even if it means going to court so a judge can tell me that I am the issue not the facility."

159

"Well that is your decision to make and maybe you should think about going somewhere else to work. Sometimes people need to go somewhere else in order to jump start them again on their career."

I just looked sat there not believing what I was hearing. Then I asked her for the list of people promoted over me like she told me she was going to bring. She made or should I say she stated that they (who ever they are) felt that there was no reason to share that information with me. What a fucking joke! Like I did not already know who was promoted over me in the facility. I sometimes cringe, laugh, and even feel downright angry at the so call leaders that management chose to promote over me. Especially when I see what kind of job they do or should I say in most cases don't do. That was about the end of the meeting for me, and it also would be the last time I would even think about seeking help from the so call AA agency.

EVEN THOUGH I HAVE BEEN told by different people to go to the Out Reach clinic on the old Griffiss Air force base, it took a long time before I went there mainly because I did not want anything to do with the military anymore. It seemed that I was in a cycle of just going to my psychiatrist just to get my medication scripts refilled. She told me that there was nothing that could be done about my night mares. I was stable, well I was more in control or should I say more not out of control. I still had issues on a regular basic. I missed talking to a therapist and I knew that I needed to speak to someone, and I could not think of anyone that I could be totally honest with. Better to talk to strangers then someone you might know. Things seem to flow more smoothly. So I finally went to the Out Reach Center and filled out the paper work, and was told that someone would call me to set up an appointment. A couple weeks later I received a call from the Syracuse VA Hospital and was asked if I did not mind going to Syracuse instead of Rome because they had a shortage of help in the Rome Clinic. I did not want to wait to be seen in Rome so I accepted the appointment in Syracuse.

In order to be seen by a psychiatrist or therapist with the VA I had to be assessed by the VA medical doctor. Most of the documentation that the other psychiatrist had on me was already in the VA system since I applied for disability a few months back. The doctor was a very polite and easy to talk to guy. We chatted about fishing and kayaking when I was there and I became so comfortable with him that I asked for him to be my regular doctor. He orders me some Prazosin HCL 10mg, which is for high blood pressure but told me it has also been known to help with nightmares. He told me I would receive the medication in the mail, and then he sent me to get my blood work done and off I went.

Next I received a phone call from a psychiatrist and set up a meeting. He seemed like a friendly sort and seems to always smile when I was with him. He was also going to put me on the Prazosin HCL as well but was surprised at how large of a dose that the MD put me on. He gave me some more scripts of my old medications and the only change was the Bupropion (generic for wellburtin). Seems the VA does not allow 300mg of Bupropion at one time and he change the order to read 150mg twice a day. I set up my next appointment and off I went.

I was surprise at how organized the VA was; hell it went against any dealings that I have had with them in the past. I guess the computer age made a lot of things easier. All of my appointments and medications were accessible to any of them. Receiving the medication in the mail was a little more work because I was only getting a months supply instead of three months. The fact that I did not have to pay any co-pays on any medications that had to deal with a service connected issue was a bonus.

Next I received a call for an appointment with a therapist. She was also a polite person, someone who I quickly became comfortable with. She was new to the VA and did not understand a lot of the military language and jobs, or how things worked in the service but lacked nothing in her confidence to do her job. We started seeing each other every week. It was something that I knew I needed. Of course she had the good me, I would laugh at her and tell her that I have come along way in the last couple years and that most of the hard work was done and I just needed some fine tuning. She laughed.

Of course she asked that all important question about me thinking about hurting myself and if I ever tried. I smiled and said that if I had I would not be here now. Of course she asked what I meant and I told her that I owned a 44 and if I attempted it I would not fail because it makes a very big hole. I did tell her that I had thought of it even had the loaded pistol to my head but I did not attempt it. I always found a reason to make it to another day. She offered me some trigger locks and I laughed at her and said what good that would do? She told me she wanted me to give one key to someone I trusted and to freeze the other one in a glass of water. She asked me if I understood why she wanted me to do this and I laughed. I said if I have to ask someone for a key or if I had to wait till the key thawed out it would give me some extra time to think about what I was doing and maybe, just maybe it would be long enough for me to change my mind. She said that is right, but I declined the locks.

The nightmares got a lot worse when I first started taking the Prazosin HCL. I kept on taking them as prescribed though. It took about three weeks before things finally settled down. Then I could not believe it the nightmares just seem to vanish. It took awhile before I would let myself believe it but it was true. I even got to the point where I would not even think or worry about me falling asleep. As far as the amount of sleep that I was getting, that did not change that much. I just got used to only getting three hours of sleep a night.

I regularly saw my therapist, and she would always give me some homework to do. Nothing like actual work, rather she would try to get me to think about what was my trigger when I became agitated. It was a good concept, because it did make me think a little clearer. I even started driving slower. Cruz control nice and slow and you know what, driving slower was really relaxing to me. I tried not to think about all the people passing me. Who cares, because I was finding out that I could go from here to there with out losing my wits?

Now my therapist wanted me to go to this new program. It was designed to try and get all that stuff that one kept hidden out in the open in an controlled environment. I did not know if I was ready to open that box but I was willing to try anything to better myself and my life. She asked me to think about it even though I told her I would do it. Three visits to her after that and I asked her if she had put me in for it and she said she had not yet and I asked her not to. I think she agreed with this because she did not seem surprised by my request. She said she wanted to make sure I was ready for it. I thought I was. I thought the worse was over and that things could only get better. That's what I get for thinking.

I don't really know what the change was. Maybe it was my body getting used to the new medication, maybe it was because my therapist had me thinking more about everything and trying to figure out why I got so frustrated or felt so distant at times. Maybe it was because I let my guard down some. After all I was overwhelmed with the results from the help that I was getting from the VA. Why did I not go there sooner? It seemed to me like the nightmares came back slowly but the truth is that I only think that they came back slowly because I did not remember them. My wife sure knew they were back. Of course the same old question from her on what bothering me and what had changed. The only thing that changed was me screaming as I woke up. They seem to get worse and worse. My heart would be beating so fast and I would be scared out of my mind and bolt upright screaming as loud as I could.

RETIRED MSG DENNIS JAMES WILLIAMS

This was why I asked my therapist not to put me in for that new program. I thought maybe I was going to fast because I had opened up a lot more to her then I have to anyone else so far. To me it is kind of hard to narrow down exactly what was the biggest thing that bothered me from Iraq, but I did mention a couple that stood out. Stood out, how funny is that? It seems that it is just a blob of memories that is faint but every now and then something happens, someone says something, or something triggers my memory and then there I am right back in the moment. If only it would stop there maybe I could get a handle on it, but one memory opens another memory and sometimes it is just too hard to think of something else.

I know my therapist asked me if I saw too much killing. I had to laugh at her and I even asked her what too much killing is? I mean is there a magical number of bodies and of blood and gore or headless corpses that one can see before they truly can say that they had seen too much? I don't consider myself a "Rambo" anymore. I know when we first got to our FOB my old Delta company soldiers were in a hurry to get out there and kick some ass. I would always tell them not to be in too much of a hurry and to be careful what they wished for. A month later none of them wanted to leave the FOB. How no one was killed is amazing, because they had NOD's shot off their faces as they drove down the street. They even found some bullets in their equipment when they back to their company area.

Can you guess what happened next? It had to be one way or another. Either they would have to keep getting shot at or they would have to get a little more aggressive. A little more aggressive is not the right word. They became the animal looking for their prey. The big three story building that they always got shot at from was now being shot up before anyone inside could shoot at them. Of course that building finally got destroyed by EOD. A great big boom that day and the only thing left standing was the elevator shaft. It was a fine monument for all to see. I know the soldiers all laughed about it all the time.

Well if you were one of the Anti-Coalition forces that were shooting at the Coalition Forces would you shoot at the aggressive infantry convoys or would you shoot at the less aggressive units? That is what happened when the Anti-Coalition forces would see the markings on our vehicles they seemed to steer away from them more and more. Our unit controlled our area, as much as any unit could.

We guarded and helped the locals build water plants and police headquarters just so the same ones who build it could destroy it so we would pay them to rebuild it. Funny if you think about it, sure does give one great job security.

Even though the nightmares were back and I was trying to figure things out I still wanted to move ahead. Maybe it was just too fast? When her and I spoke it was in a nice environment but our conversation always stayed with me when I left and longer. I long for the day when one can label me free of PTSD. My therapist says it will never truly fully happen. That it will always be there but the trick was to what degree. The trick was trying to put it in a place where one could function in society without standing out. I wish it was that easy. I have lots of memorable moments in the service both good and bad. It is hard to think of the good without the bad. So I have tried to erase my military history out of me. I have even told people I have never served but deep down I want to scream that I have swerved and that I am not looking for anything special but in the same token I am not the same as those who have never served.

Going to the VA has helped me with this. It has given me the strength that I needed to admit that I have some things that have left a mark on my soul and that I should not run and hide from that fact. I should embrace it and let it be a positive thing for me, at least as much as possible.

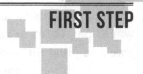

21

FIRST STEP

THE FIRST STEP OF TRYING to find me was a hard one, because I had to sever the ties that I had to the world that was keeping me going. The drugs, the alcohol, the special friend, all of them had a certain role in keeping me going to the next day but if I did not change and get away from all of them I could never be myself again. Rather I would just keep on being that thing for someone else. Maybe that would have been the case if it had not been for my daughters. My daughters were the true reason that I finally woke up and saw the light. I saw what I had become and how I affected them. I did not like what I saw and I knew that I had to change my ways.

The first step was to get away from that special friend that made my life so enjoyable to me. It was hard, to say the least. It was made easier by her actions against a new friend that I had come fond of. The lies that she had spread through many avenues to include e-mails on the work system, on Face Book, on My Space, and even word of mouth. This did cause me a lot of issues with my new friend because I kept telling her to just ignore her and that she would stop and go away. I did not want to tell her everything that went on between her and I but the more time that I spent and the closer that I got to her the more I told her.

All I can say is that you can't be friends with someone who goes out of their way and knowingly tries to make things harder for you. How sad is this? We could have stayed friends; we could have been there for one another for years to come. Of course some of the things we did would have to stop, but our relationship had grown way beyond sex. At least in my mind it did. I think that in her mind she was losing much more than I was. I think she saw me as her steady rock. I had up to this point put her ahead of everything and everyone. Any problem that she had for the last couple of years was handled by me and not by her husband. My wife always complained of this and I just ignored it because I was alive when I did her biddings.

Yes she was on the way out. There was no movement forward for me without this step. It was a long drawn out step but it was in the process of being made. Of course it is hard to just quit cold turkey. So I found myself being drawn back to her with excuses of what was going on. We both knew that things had changed and we both saw what was happening. She kept using the crutches that she had on me to keep me longer then I should have stayed. They only worked, could only work for so little of a time. I had stopped living for her and was looking for that path to find me.

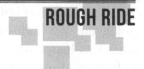

22

ROUGH RIDE

SOONER OR LATER EVERYONE OR everyone catches up to either some one or something I was no different and I too finally caught up with myself. It was a close call in more ways then one. With all the drinking, smoking, snorting, and spending nights who knows where something was bound to happen. Of course I was not thinking at all and if I was in my state back then I most likely would not have cared. I most likely would have welcomed the outcome with open arms. Trying to spend time with the old friend to keep her happy and yet spend time with the new friend to keep her happy and to try and do other things in my life finally caught up to me. Of course the fact that I was not sleeping much might have had something to do with it. I would always drive on the seat of my pants either from the road rage or from the fight to keep my eyes awake. On this day I lost. On this day the odds finally gripped me with both arms and hugged me tightly.

I left at five in the morning from my latest friend's house and started off to my camp. My camp had become my get away from everything. It was a place where I always feel comfortable and at ease. My grandfather built it in 1961 and I had acquired it from my mother just a few short years ago. I was in the process of remodeling everything in it and around it. I enjoyed the work, which I never called work but more of a hobby. Of course the camp was way out in no mans land of Tug Hill, so there is no cell phone service.

Well I was driving there and I was feeling good. Radio was not blaring but it was a little on the loud side. I went by Burger King and thought of getting some breakfast. Maybe it would give me some energy to keep me going. Normally I do stop but on this day I did not have a lot of extra money so I decided to save what little I had for some gas so I kept driving,

All of a sudden I felt a little bump and had just enough time to open my eyes to see the wire guards right in front of me. I attempted to pull away but once the front of the truck hit the wires it was all over. The wire seem to hold me on their path and I skirted down thirty feet or so of it before I could get it off the wire. I did not have anytime to be scared and I remember it like it was yesterday and the fact that I was not even worried about the damage to the truck. I was thankful that I was unhurt. I pulled over to the other side of the road just past the guard wires and tried to get out of the truck. The door was jammed but after a couple good hard thrust with my shoulder it sprung free. I got out and said "shit!" I just noticed that I had three flat tires. I had just put four new tires on the truck only two weeks ago and now I got three flats. Funny that the fact that I had just bought all four tires and how I wasted 500 dollars was the thing that bothered me the most about the accident Shit what do you do now? No traffic, no cell service.

I scanned the area and tried to place where I was on the road. One of my co-workers lived up the road, and although I did not know how far it was to me it was the logical way to go. So off I went on my nice hike that turned out to be just over a mile. When I got there I banged on her front door hoping I could get an answer from someone so I could use the phone. Nothing, all was quiet and still.

Shit I said, and looked around. I knew her mother and father lived right next door to her and although I did not know them it is the place I headed to next. When I got on the porch I could see movement in the house and I was immediately surprised and glad. I knocked on the door and her mother approached it and then stopped ten feet away and called for her husband. I guess that the fact that a stranger was knocking on the door at five thirty in the morning would be enough to make anyone worry, but the fact that I had shoulder length purple hair must have took her back some also. I heard her called to her husband and I told her that I worked with her daughter and called her by name, and that I had had a accident and needed to use a phone. When she heard me call her daughter's name she opened the door and welcomed me in. She had me sit at the dinning room table and offered me some breakfast. I declined the breakfast but accepted some orange juice. Her mother and father sat down and talked with me, seems her mother was busy making supper. That's right I said supper. Who gets up that early to make supper? Wonder if John Boy is around, you know Walton's Mountain.

Anyway I called 911 and was told to wait where I was until the sheriff arrived. It was better then walking back anyway. After that I called my father, even though it was forty miles away he got out of bed and drove out to get me. The Deputy Sheriff arrived and boy was she a looker, young and hot and in uniform with a gun, my dream come true. She of course asked what happened, and like a good honest citizen of the United States I told her exactly what happened when those deer ran out in the road. LOL. You do not think I told her that I dozed off now do you. Hell she might give me a ticket for crossing a double yellow line or something. Oh that is right I could get that anyway, because it does not matter why you crossed the line just that you did. Oh well guess there is worse things then to get a ticket.

"You have to sit in the back seat because my front seat is full." She said as we were leaving.

"Are you going to handcuff me?"

"No, why would I do that you are not under arrest?"

"Being arrested is not the only reason to put handcuffs on someone."

She stopped and looked at me and I could see the smile on her face. Maybe it was a little forward but hell it felt so right to say it. I hopped in the car and off we went. Of course I kept talking to her, nothing seductive or anything, just about the area and how her day was going.

When we got to the scene of the accident she said that I was very lucky. It seems the wire rail had stopped my truck from going over a sharp decline down twenty feet into a swap / pond. I never really noticed that when I pulled over. Now every time I go by the place I smile and think of the accident. I smile about it, because I know I was very lucky that day. Hell a car could have been coming the other way and I would of smash into them head on. Yup it could have been a lot worse.

She called for a flat bed and waited with me. Would be nice to tell you a wild story of what happened at this time between the sheriff and me but that would not be true. We chatted until the flatbed truck arrived. The driver pulled in front and started loading my truck just as my father arrived. We made arrangements for him to deliver the truck to a collision place in my home town. He said it would be a couple days and I just laughed because I had no choice and I did not think I would be driving it any time soon. Good thing I had a summer rat to drive. My summer rat was a car I bought to save money on gas. Seems the payment was less then what I saved on gas. Love my Dodge but it sure drinks a lot.

The sheriff left and the flatbed truck driver made a comment about her not giving me a ticket. Seems she usually does not let anyone get away without a ticket. I laughed and told him what I said to her about the cuffs and maybe she got a chuckle out of it that she let me go. We all laughed over this and then my truck was carried away and my father drove me home.

A week later the insurance company assessor came out and totaled my truck because of the amount of cosmetic damage to it. I asked him about how much I would get and he said around ten thousand dollars. I was relieved because of how much I was getting since the truck was all paid for. It got even better when I was able to buy it back from them for a thousand dollars. I then received a check for $10,400.00. WOW! It cost me $3,500 to fix my truck so that it was legal to run on the road. I needed three new tires, a new rim, a new front bumper and quarter panel. Still it left me with a good chunk of change, so I bought each one of my kids a new lab top.

I had to take the truck to Syracuse to a DMV shop to have it inspected. They had to check the serial numbers for the new parts and also the fact that it had been fixed. Seems they check the serial numbers to hamper car thieves from scrapping vehicles. Then I was given a new title, well it was not a new title it was a savage title. Cost me $200.00, but it was worth it because later when I was going through a divorce my wife tried to get some money for the truck and I laugh and said it was not worth anything because it had a salvage title. Believe it or not it worked. One time I got the better hand then her.

23

BUMPS IN THE ROAD

THE ROAD TO ANYWHERE IS never straight, it always has curves and some bumps here and there. After all if it was straight what fun would that be? So was the road to self discovery and self control. Every now and then something would happen to test you and keep you on your toes. Sometimes just dealing with people is enough to make you wonder if you can handle yourself all the time or not. You know you got those people who think they are better then you or better then the law. As a matter of fact I ran into one of those people.

It was a nice relaxing day and my youngest daughter and I were driving to the shopping mall to return some sneakers that I had purchased on line for her, because they sent sneakers with men sizes instead of ladies. Would it not be easier to just have one set size for everyone?

Anyway I was driving and I came to a traffic light. The light was green but there were two cars in front of me with their blinkers on turning left. They were hugging the middle of the road and there was plenty of room on their right to get past. I did not think anything of it. Even when I seen the county sheriff car near the intersection I did not think anything was wrong. All of a sudden the sheriff's car pulled out into the intersection some. I slowed down and waited to see where he was going. I even made a comment to my daughter about his actions.

When he stopped I kept going around the cars and continued on my way. Of course he flew around the corner and turned his lights on. SHIT! Ok I will admit maybe it was a bad move on my part, but in my defense I did not see him until I was alongside the other cars and so I just went on my way. To the sheriff he might have thought that I was being disrespectful to him. Maybe this even ticked him off some but he is exposing to be a professional and should not let his agitation at someone he pulls over show.

Well he approached my stopped car and asked for my licenses, registration and proof of insurance. I asked him if there was something wrong and he said to give me my licenses and registration and then he would tell me. I got my licenses and registration out but had a hard time finding my current proof of insurance. I had an older one so I gave that to him and told him that it was the same policy and that I could not find the other one. He then told me that I crossed a hazard line when I passed those two cars on the right, and asked me, no rather shouted at me that that was why he pulled out in front of me and did I not see him.

At this time I was holding my own pretty good. He checked out the registration, must have seen my corrections union sticker on the window but that was not going to help me today. He asked me where I lived and I told him my address, he told me to tell him again slowly so he could write it down. I should have been smart enough to not tell him where I lived but the address on my licenses. I had my PO Box still on my licenses even though I had reported my change to the DMV. The DMV told me that the place where I get my mail is what is exposing to be on my licenses. I tried to explain this to the officer but all he wanted was the information that he asked for and was not listening to anything that I was saying. Of well I guess I am going to get a ticket.

Fifteen minutes . . . twenty minutes . . . thirty minutes . . . forty minutes. What the fuck is he doing? Of course by this time I am getting a little more agitated then I wanted. I tried to do as my therapist says and try to focus on my triggers and try to calm myself down. Of course I am talking or complaining to my self now. What the fuck can he be doing? Every time I look back there it seems like he is picking up and setting down the same piece of paper. When it hit an hour and he was still in his car I could not sit still anymore and I got out of my car. He yelled for me to get back in my car but it was too late for me to listen to him. I yelled at him to fuck-off and proceeded to get out and pace in front of my car. Fifty feet down the side of the road and back again. Over and over I paced for another ten minutes. I then turned around and he was standing at my car. As I was approaching back to the car he told me to take all day that he did not care because he was getting paid.

I got back into my car and said to him that waiting for an hour to get a ticket was fucking ridiculous. I looked at all the tickets that he was carrying and asked him how many tickets he was giving me? Five he said. Five, what the fuck did I do to deserve five tickets. He then read them off to me

173

1. Crossing a hazard marker.
2. Going off the pavement to pass.
3. No proof of insurance.
4. Failure to notify DMV of address change.
5. Failure to notify DMV of registration address change.

Just give me the fucking tickets and let me go on my way. You would think that at this time it would be best for both of us to part ways. No he has to keep on and he went so far as to tell me he would pull me out of my car. Of course the only thing he was getting from me at this time is to fuck off and that he was an asshole. He tried to get me to threaten him so that he could have an excuse to put his hands on me and stated to me that everything was being taped. He then stated that he could yank me out of my car if he wishes. I laughed at him and said I do not think so. Most people would be intimated by an officer of the law especially if one was acting the way that this one was. Maybe if I would have just said yes sir and no sir would have been better for me. Who the fuck does he think he is that he could harass me in the name of justice and that I would just sit there and take it. He has got the wrong boy that is for sure.

Of course he did not give me the tickets. He proceeded to take his time and read everyone to me as I am screaming to him to just give me my fucking tickets and calling him an ass hole. Ten more minutes this went on with me screaming at him before he finally gave me my tickets and licenses back. I threw them into the car and call him another name and that it was ridiculous to have to wait so fucking long. He just smiled and told me to pull out slowly and I just told him to fuck off again and that he was an ass hole.

The tickets that the Officer gave me had me going to court on Sunday 9/23/2012. When I got there the building seemed deserted. I tried every door and then went to the police station behind the court house, where again I did not get any answer. I left and returned the next day to the court secretary who told me that court was not held on Sundays, and that it was held only on Tuesdays. I showed her the tickets with the date of Sunday 9/23/2012. She asked me what I wanted to do with the tickets and I told her I wanted to talk to the District Attorney. She had me make a plea of not guilty and gave me a packet and to write to the District Attorney.

So I wrote to the county district attorney and explained what had transpired as I remembered it.

To: County District Attorney's Office
Re: #12090118.01-.05

Re:	Case No.	Statute/Section	Description:	Ticket No.
	12090118.01	VTL 1123 OB	Passing Violation	312200WFDF
	12090118.02	VTL 1128 D	CHG Lane Hazard	312200WGDF
	12090118.03	VTL 0319 01U	Insurance Violation	312200WHDF
	12090118.04	VTL 0401 03	Registration Violation	312200WKDF
	12090118.05	VTL 0509 08	FL NTFY ADD CHG	312200WLDF

QUESTIONS ON INSTRUCTIONS SHEET:	ANSWER
1. Was there an accident?	1. NO
2. Acknowledgment of liability	2. N/A
3. Do you have a criminal record?	3. NO
4. Any prior or pending alcohol related offenses?	4. NO
5. Any pending charge in another court?	5. NO

Dear County District Attorney,

I Dennis Williams would like to explain how I feel that it was an injustice on the part of the Officer to have issued me these five tickets listed above. I would first like to explain a little about myself in the attempt that some of my actions might be understood a little better. I am a retired disabled veteran with 24 years of service and two combat tours. I have a 40% disability and am dealing with PTSD and all of the frustrating symptoms of it.

On the said date of September 3, 2012 I was taking my daughter to the Destiny Center mall to return some wrong size sneakers that I had order for her through the mail. I was not speeding and we were enjoying our time together. I came to the intersection of Route 31 and Torchwood lane and the light was green but there were two cars in front of me who were turning left. The traffic was congested quite a bit. I slowed down to almost a crawl and proceeded to go around them on the right. I do admit that my right side tires did go across the white line but I never left the pavement at any time.

As I was going around the cars I noticed the sheriff's car at the intersection, but thought nothing of it. The officer pulled the front of his car forward from the stopping point. I stopped to let the Officer go where ever it was that he was trying to go. The Officer stopped and after a moment I continued on my way. He immediately pulled around the corner and put his lights on to pull me over. I proceeded to turn my turn signal on and pulled to the shoulder of the road.

The Officer approached my car and asked for my licenses and registration and proof of insurance. I asked him if there was anything wrong and he said he would tell me after I gave him what he asked for. I got my registration and my licenses but had a hard time finding a current insurance card, but I found one that had just run out and handed it to him and stated that it did not have the right dates but that it was the same policy.

The Officer told me he pulled me over for crossing a hazard line and asked if I saw him or not pulling out in the intersection in front of me. I told him I did and that I did not know what he was doing and after he stopped I proceeded on my way. I can see how someone might think that I was being disrespectful and rude to them but I assure you that was not the case. I was already around the cars and it did not seem to be a choice but to continue on my way.

The Officer then asked me where I lived and I told him my address. He asked me to say it again slower because it was not written on any of the information that I had given him. He then asked me how long I lived there and if I had notifies DMV of the address change. I told him eight months and yes I did notify the DMV of my address change and that there was nothing wrong with my licenses.

He then went back to his car. I sat there trying to patiently wait for him; I started to get a little frustrated after thirty-five minutes. Every time I looked back he was sitting there and I could not understand what could possibly be taking so long. After an hour I was too frustrated and I knew that I had to unwind myself so I did not lose control. I got out of my car to pace in front of it, I heard the Officer shout out of his car but I do not know what he said and I continued out in front of my car, where I paced up and down the road about fifty feet for another ten minutes. I turned around and he was standing at my car. He told me "take your time I got all day and I am getting paid".

I got back in my car and stated that waiting an hour to get a ticket is fucking ridicules. The Officer stated to me that everything was being taped and I told him I did not care. The Officer made a couple more comments to me and it seemed like he was trying to get me to say something threatening to him, but I did not. Around this time the Officer threatened to pull me out of my car. I told him that I did not think so. I then saw the bunch of tickets in his hand and asked him how many tickets he was giving me. He stated five and I said five what could I possible have done to receive five tickets. The Officer stated what the tickets were for and I laughed at him and said again that there was nothing wrong with my licenses. I then asked him for my tickets and he just took his time and started to read every ticket to me. I shouted for him to just give me my tickets and he refused to. He seemed to take his time and took another five minutes just reading the tickets to me.

He then gave me the tickets and my information back to me. My licenses dropped beside my left said and I tried to open the door to retrieve it. The Officer pushed my door closed and when I told him what I was doing he said he did not care and for me to get it later. He then told me to pull out slowly and I left.

The ticket that the Officer gave me had me going to court on Sunday 9/23/2012. When I got there the building seemed deserted. I tried every door and then went to the police station behind the court house, where again I did not get any answer. I left and returned the next day to the court secretary who told me that court was not held on Sundays, and that it was held only on Tuesdays. I showed her the tickets with the date of Sunday 9/23/2012. She asked me what I wanted to do with the tickets and I told her I wanted to talk to the District Attorney. She had me make a plea of not guilty and gave me a packet and to write to the District Attorney.

On case number 12090118.03 about statute VTL 0319 01U dealing with an Insurance Violation on ticket number 312200WHDF I have enclosed a copy of my current insurance card that shows that I have proper insurance on said vehicle at the time of the incident.

On case number 12090118.04 about statute VTL 0401 03 dealing with a Registration Violation on ticket number 312200WKDF are untrue because I did notify DMV of my change of address but I get my mail at the PO Box and I was told by DMV that the PO Box is the one to go on the registration of the vehicle.

On case number 12090118.05 about statue VTL 0509 08 dealing with Failure to Notify DMV of Address Change on ticket number 312200WLDF are untrue because as stated before I did notify DMV of my change of address but I get my mail at the PO Box and I was told by DMV that the PO Box is the one to go on my licenses.

On case number 12090118.01 about statue VTL 1123 OB on Leaving the Pavement to pass on ticket number 312200WFDF is untrue because I never left the pavement.

On case number 12090118.02 about statue VTL 1128 D on Changing Lane Hazard on ticket number 312200WGDF I concede that I did cross the white hazard line but I request that it be thrown out due to the improper way that the

Officer treated me. At the scene the Officer was very unprofessional, and the situation could have escalated because of his actions and comments to me. By giving me a court date when he must have known the court was closed only go to prove my case that the Officer was unprofessional and maybe even a little spiteful.

If you don't agree that my opinion of the events and the proof I sent to you is enough to throw the tickets out I respectfully request a copy of the tape that the Officer stated to me was being recorded.

Sincerely,

When the District Attorney finally wrote back to me they informed me that if I was found guilty on all tickets it would be eight points on my licenses. They offered me a deal with pleading guilty to just the failure to notify DMV of a address change. I had to smile at this because it was one of the tickets that was surely bogus. As much as I wanted to get this officer in front of the judge I knew that it would be in my best interest to take the deal, so I pleaded guilty on the form and mailed it back to the courts. Now I just await my fine, and I do not get any points on my licenses.

24

GOODBYE FLIGHT

EVERYONE HAS HIS OR HER first true love. The one who magically made you feel like you were on the top of the world and no one could touch you. Well I had my first true love long ago when I was in high school. Just like anyone else she was everything to me and the short time we spent together lasted me a life time. Two weeks after high school I left for Fort Benning to become one of America's finest infantrymen. Better then that I was on my way to becoming one of America's paratroopers.

I asked her if she wanted to break our relationship off when I left. I thought it would be easier on her, and I was pleasantly surprised when she said no, and that she would wait for me. I can still see her tears flowing down her face as that Grey Hound bus drove away. We did try to keep in touch and stay close but like that saying goes "Jody got your girl back home," he took mine and she was gone. For me it was easy to stay true, because she was always with me. She was always on my mind and always in my heart.

Twenty-four years later and I am signed up to a web site that has your high school reunions on it and I look one day and I have a message from her. I was nervous and afraid to open it but I also was excited. It was just a friendly letter asking if I remembered her. Remembered her? How could she ask such a question? I wrote back to her and told her how I never stopped loving her and how she was always on my mind.

We were just friends talking about our lives to each other and it felt good to have someone listen. This went on for a couple months and then she asked me not to contact her anymore as her husband was having a hard time with her talking to me. I agreed and did as she requested, but I told her I would always be here if she needed me. I did keep all of our emails in a folder that I read now and then.

The next time that I heard from her she was divorced. It was a quick divorce if ever there was one. Again we started to chat again on the computer. It was a much-needed escape from my living hell that I was trying to figure out. Surely this could only complicate things more. We had some good conversations at least in my mind we did. I did a search and got her address and her phone number. I was going to surprise her. SURPRISE! It really would have been a surprise since I lived in New York and she was living in Nebraska. To me it was only a stone throw away and I wanted to see her in person.

I did tell her that I had her address and phone number and she asked what it was. I told her and she laughed, seems I got the number right but the address was the house where her and her x-husband had lived. She was a little uncomfortable with this. I tried to explain to her that to me it was only yesterday that we parted and that I wanted to be able to say my goodbyes in person. She understood this and talked about doing the same to someone in her past, and how much it helped her.

Finally after a few weeks I got her to agree to see me as long as it was when she did not have her son. I agreed and she gave me some dates when he would be with his father. I quickly called and got a flight that would of kept me in Nebraska as long as possible with the dates that she gave me. Could it really be happening, could the moment that I wanted to have for so many years finally come true?

I did not let anyone know what I was doing or where I was going. I just hopped on the plane and away I went. When my plane finally landed and I was walking out of the plane I saw her there leaning on the wall. I quickly stepped into the bathroom to freshen up before saying hello to her. I don't recall what color my hair was at this time but I know it was shoulder length long. When I finally thought I had my composure down, I walked out and said hello to her.

She asked me if I had checked a bag and I said all I got is this carry on and off we went. When we got outside where the heat hit me and I thought I was looking out at the dessert in Iraq. After a brief moment I came back to reality, or should I say as much of a reality as could be expected because it sure felt like a dream rather then the present. With all the flash backs and memories it still was hard at times knowing the difference between what was real and what was going on only in my mind.

She must have noticed something in me because she said something to me. I tried very hard not to show any emotions but after she spoke it was too much for me to bear and the tears just started to flow like a river. I wiped my eyes as well as I could and told her not to mind the tears and that I had longed for this day since I left for the Army back in July of 1982. The sight of her and her tears in my mother's car as the Greyhound bus pulled away on that day still is as vivid today in my mind as it was back then. If ever there was any happiness in my childhood it was with her. She had made me feel like I was someone special and I would of done anything for her. I still smile when ever I see one of those many moments in my mind.

It did not take long to get to her apartment and when we got settled down on the couch we both brought out our yearbooks from High School and exchanged with one another. It was kind of nice to read the things that were said long . . . long . . . long ago. It was like a walk down memory lane where we spoke of and laughed at the silly things that we did. We played some cards and went out to eat. I went to bed early as the emotional drain as well as the flight left me exhausted. I did not sleep in the same bed or room as her. I slept in her son's bed. I never pushed toward anything besides the fact that she has always been on mine in one way or another and I wanted to put closer finally on the dream that I once lived.

I wished we could have hit it off like old friends but there was a difference between us. I know this because I could sense that we both felt it. The first day was nice and the second day alright but by the third day we were grasping at things to do or talk about. I know this hurt me a lot to finally realize that I was just a young boyfriend of hers and that the importance of our relationship so far ago was cherished more by me then by her. Maybe when she wrote to me at first it was because she was trying to deal with her own issues and she never really expected me to answer.

When it was time to go she drove me back to the airport and dropped me off in front of the terminal. It was an awkward goodbye and I attempted to give her a hug and she pulled away. I was a little shocked and hurt. I was with her for three days and did not try anything and all I was attempting to do was get a farewell hug. I shrugged it off and turned and walked away never looking back to see if she watch me walk away or drove quickly away. It did not matter because I had achieved what I had thought about for all those years. I finally got to say goodbye.

A big snow storm had hit Chicago and all of the airplanes out to there were cancelled. I spent that night on the floor of the terminal. Not once did I even think of calling her. I was not upset; I was more like in recovery from the emotional release from the weekend. I did end up getting put on another plane somewhere in the middle of the night. I could still make my connecting flight in Chicago, I guess sometimes having a long layover helps. Nope! Even though the airport in Chicago was running all of the cancelled flights had a rippling effect. The flights that were scheduled to take off were almost all full and the people from the cancelled flight were put on a waiting list according to the airlines rules. I was number six and the next flight was in the next morning. I called worked to tell them that I would not be in tomorrow and maybe longer.

Chicago O'Hare airport really was not that big but it was very busy and there was people laying everywhere from all the cancelled flights. You had to be lucky to find any room now, but I was lucky there was a USO there. I walked in and sat down. Some guy called me over and said that the room was only for military personnel. When I told him I was retired he asked for my military identification card, which I quickly showed him. Maybe it was the long colored hair that made me look out of place. He made a comment about the card and I could feel his approach to me change. I bet he never would have guessed that I was a MSG.

I sat down again and looked around the room. It was not much but to a traveling military person it was like an oasis in the dessert. They had free coffee, juice and some Danishes to eat. There were four computers set up, and a big screen television on. They also had a back small room with some cots but they were all full. I tried to make myself as comfortable as I could in the chair and closed my eyes. It was not a very good sleep more like a haze, where I was watching the television but where I had no idea what was going on. More like a distraction from everything, keeping my mind from wandering on its own.

Not only was it a little bit more homely but I also put in to be woken up before my flight time so I did not have to worry about oversleeping. I got to the flight gate and had to wait like everyone else. I did not have to go to see anyone until I was called and I could see my name on the standing list. It was five minutes before take off time and I was still three on the list. I could hear others complaining and leave to get breakfast. I had no where else to go so I sat there waiting for my name. Two minutes before scheduled take off time I heard the called for the two people that just left. I looked all over to see them and smiled when I did not. Soon I heard my name and I approached the gate. I had just enough time to walk to the back of the plane and sit down before it started to taxi to the runway.

When I landed in Syracuse airport I finally could let what had just transpired over the last four days start to sink in. I knew that I would have to answer some questions from my new girlfriend. I could have lied and come up with this fantastic story but I chose to tell the truth and let things take care of them selves. I explained that I went to say goodbye to my long last girlfriend and that I did not tell her because I knew she would tell me if I went that it would be over between us and that I still would have chosen to go. Of course this did not go over very well and a big fight broke out. She could not understand what I was attempting to do and all she saw was me flying all over the country to meet a girl.

Something was different inside of me, and I knew I was at peace with our past. It is kind of hard to explain but it was like this emptiness was gone. Like a hole filled in. Nothing was left to fall into. Even though it hurt to know I was not as important to her as she was to me, in the end it did not matter because she did mean that much to me and nothing could take that away.

25

A SPECIAL FRIEND

As I SAID BEFORE I was living for and through someone else. I started to realize this more and more. I started to question myself as to what I was doing and what I was losing. I knew that I had to change something. Unfortunately I was still not able to stand on my own. Although if you would of asked me then I would of said sure with no problem. The more that I noticed that our relationship was not what it once was, or better yet what I perceived it to be, and that I could never really be totally happy and secure in it, the more I started to try and find a new path.

Things just sort of work them selves out sometime. In this case I got some information third hand about someone. The information sort of got my mind wondering. I won't say what it was that I learned or how I learned it out of respect for her. Because of this information I wanted to get to talk to someone that I never have spoken to before. My chance came shortly after learning about them. Maybe it was because I was looking for away to get closer without being so blunt as to say "hello how you doing". Someone wanted a swap (working someone else's shift in exchange they work one for you). Me being able to work any schedule because of the way that I was living made it easy to go out of my way for them.

In the course of getting the paper work for the swap done I took the opportunity to ask them a few questions. Maybe it was a little forward of me but I just played it as if I was just curious and that I meant no harm. I am sure it got them wondering what my motives were. Something she would tell me later on.

Then I noticed that she was on MY Space every night. So I started to send her quick little notes. You know like how you doing, why are you up so late, how was work. Of course this led to other conversations and soon we were chatting most every night and into the morning. She would ask me what I was looking for and I would say nothing really just needed someone to talk to. She said that she did not believe me and that I was not going to get in her pants. Well even if I had ideas of doing just that I told her ok and that I just needed a friend. Of course I don't think she believed me but I also think she was enjoying my company as much as I was enjoying hers.

She kept telling me that nothing was going to happen physically between us. I kept telling her that I did not care, and that I just wanted a friend. It was not just a friend that I was looking for, but I was enjoying having someone who I could talk to especially since she was not involved in my life in any way. Kind of like a referee, asking me those questions that I failed to focus on even though I knew they were there.

It started out as just chatting and then I went to her friend's house to play some cards, and have a few beers. It was a nice relaxing and enjoyable time with no stress at all. I did as I said I would do and did not try anything with her. She seemed to be worried about this but after a couple times going out she seemed to not mention it as much. With all the drama that was going on in my life it was nice to actually have a real friend just to chat with. Of course she got a friend in return and she was dealing with her own issues. I never tried to be her night in shining armor, but I was there for her if she needed me to be.

Things changed on a specific night that we were out playing cards and drinking. She got a little over drunk if ever there was a word for that. Bombed, plastered, what ever you want to call it. I did not think she was that far gone, she was a little giggle, maybe even a little flirty but I was sticking by my word. Even when one of our friends' there made a comment to me that she did not hear. I shook my head no. I had no intentions of trying something with her just because she was not fully aware of what was going on, I mean who would do that? Funny I know most would of, but I did not.

Now the problem came when I was driving her home and turned down her street. She told me to stop like there was something going on so I did. She jumped across the seat and attacked me with her mouth. I was a little taken off guard but I did not lose my composure. I did get her back on the other side of the seat and started driving again, though I had to stop because she attacked me again. It was nice and I surely did not want to stop but I did as I told her I would do when we first started talking. I was a stand up guy, in more ways then one. I took her home and left.

The next day she called me and very shyly asked if she could ask me a question. Of course I said anything. Then she asked me if we kissed and I laughed at her.

"Kissed hell we jumped in the back seat don't you remember?"

"We did not I would remember that."

"Well I don't think you remembered all that had happened last night if you have to ask me if we kissed."

"Stop playing Dennis and tell me the truth."

"Yes you attacked me on the way home and we kissed but I did as you asked and stopped us from doing anything more. I did not want you mad at me the next day. I would not do that to you. I stopped you from doing anything more."

Things went on as if nothing happened that night. I chalked it up to too much alcohol and was glad I did the right thing. Of course the next time we were out drinking and I took her home I did the right thing as well. She was not as drunk as she was on the other occasion and seemed fully in control of herself. We had a fun night and off I went to my other world.

The next day she e-mails me and says she does not want to hang around with me anymore. I was dumbfounded. I asked her why not and I had to chuckle at her reply. Seems she was upset that I have not tried anything with her and she was feeling a little rejected. I laughed and told her I was doing as she stated she wanted me to do in the beginning and that the next time I would be a little more attentive to her.

The next time came at a small gathering at her friend's house. The gathering was just the three of us. We sat on the porch listening to some music, had a few drinks and watched the stars and the cars go by. When her friend decided it was a night we left. I asked her where she wanted to go and she said she did not care. I told her not to tell me that because if she did I would take her to a hotel, and again she said she did not care.

So off we went right to where I said I would take her. I won't go into the hot details but I will say that we both had a great time and that we both fell asleep in each other's arms. Of course I did not care but she did, she was married and even though she and her husband were living apart she was still worried of what he would say or do. I told her to relax and just tell him that she fell asleep at her friend's house. She got dressed in a hurry and told me to get off the bed that she had to go. I started to laugh and told her that she should put her pants on the right way if she wants any kind of story to be believed. Seems she had them inside out, and we did get a big laugh out of that, both then and now.

I took her back to her friend's house and we pounded on the door until she woke up. She called her husband from her house phone and said she was sorry and that she was on her way home since he was at the house watching the kids. When she got home he was right there with the questions for her on what happened last night. She did have a good story to tell him even if it was not like her to do anything like that. As she walked in and saw him all she could do is laugh. I guess there really was not much for her to say to him after all. I bet he looked and felt dumbfounded and silly by her actions. After that night in the hotel room things just sort of took off for us.

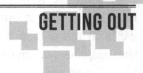

26

WHAT EVER CHANGED INSIDE OF me also took away my old desires to do just about anything, especially anything to do with hunting and fishing. The two things that I loved to do above all else. After all it does not get any calmer then when you are sitting in a tree stand on a nice warm fall afternoon. Some of my most peaceful times are when I am all alone with myself and nature. With all the issue that I was either trying to deal with or trying to avoid having the time to do anything was hard enough, but it was not just the time, I had no desire to do anything. Maybe this was one of the issues that I had to change, finding time for myself, my old self.

Alone comes Larry, a co-worker on my assigned ward, he is always fun and enjoyable to work with. He wanted to go fishing but he had no equipment, I told him that I would take him and that he did not need anything that I had everything. Well Larry is a little stubborn on a lot of things and using someone else fishing pole was one of these. I told him if he wanted his own to go buy some and explained to him to get a reel with six or more ball bearings. He was unsure of what to get so I told him I would take him to Bass Pro Shop. I told him that it would be the best place for fishing gear, but the only store in New York is in Auburn which is almost two hours away. Larry told me he did not care and that he had five hundred dollars in his pocket for me to spend on him. So we set a date. It was my first of many dates with Larry.

We met up and drove to the store. It was a very slow and nerve racking ride to the store. I don't want to knock anyone who takes care of their belongings. To say that Larry thought of his truck as his baby is just an understatement. It is almost paid for and only has 30,000 miles and it not only looks new but also smells new. How the hell does someone do that? Well Larry does not drive over the speed limit which is good in some aspects but when he got behind a tractor trailer on the New York State Thruway I finally had to say something. I asked him if he could at least pass the truck and stated that it was the most dangerous place to drive. Of course the fact that I can't handle being behind something I can not see over or around. It was nice of him to at least do this for me.

When we got to the store we went directly over to the fishing area but stopped short at the fish tank. After pointing out some of the fishes and their names and how they position themselves in the water and how to fish for them when they are on the bottom, top, or around some kind of structure. Larry was explaining to me how he fish off a boat with another co-worker who would troll for walleye. I explained to Larry that there was many ways to fish and everyone has their own favorite way, and that I was going to set him off to fish for most of them, but that if he ever is walking through a store and he sees some kind of fishing lure or something that catches his eye to buy it and to try it out. I later had to recant my directions when he told me he bought a spool of 30 pound monofilament line. I guess he did not want that big one to get away.

"What the hell are you going to do with that?"

"You said to buy anything that caught my eye."

I chuckled to myself and said "I said any lure that caught your eye buddy."

I tried to explain as much as I could to Larry about what I was buying. We were going Bass fishing so I help him pick out some wobblers and some plastic lures. I also got him some hooks and sinkers and a bobber. We picked out two nice poles one with eight bearings and one with ten. Anybody could be a great fisherman with all the gear that we got him. We spent the entire five hundred bucks.

We decided to stop for something to eat and drink. Larry was celebrating his purchase so he had a few beers. Now as we were leaving Larry stated that he did not drink and drive and asked me if I would. Of course I had no problem with this. To me the drive back was just a normal one, but then of course I am not normal. Larry never knew it could go so fast or handle so well especially on windy, dippy roads. It would be the last time that he would allow me to drive his vehicle. We still laugh about it though. Is it not what friends do laugh at those memories that stand out for what ever reason? Memories are stitched in the brain, so they are stitched in time.

One of those most memorable moments happened on our first outing in my ten foot Crawdad flat bottom boat. We went to Cazenovia Lake, which is a small semi-private lake. There is a boat launch that you can pay to use but they only let so many non-residents in a day, but at the southern tip of the lake there is an area that people launch small boats and kayaks. This is the area that we pulled into and off loaded all our gear into the Crawdad and set out on our first fishing adventure together.

A few things happened that day one was when I came to realize that Larry was a little uneasy in the boat, which only caused me to rock it over and over again. This was funny to me and after awhile I could see Larry getting more comfortable in the boat so I stopped the trolling motor and we settled in to catch some fish. I looked at the lure that Larry had on his pole.

"What the fuck is that?" I said.

"This is my dieing side winding shad wrap, and it is illegal to use in competition in seven states! Besides what is that mess you got on your pole?"

"Well this is my eight inch white salamander and the Bass love them." I said

"Watch what my lure does." Larry said.

It only took about ten minutes of me reeling in Bass after Bass before Larry was begging me to put a white salamander on his pole. I just laughed and gave him the salamander and the hook. He showed me his puppy dog eyes and said please Dennis put it on my pole for me. So I showed him how to tie it on and rig the salamander so it was weed less. I explained to him that you could not fish it wrong. It goes on the top, you can let it sink, or you can just leave it in the water. Larry started fishing with it and BAM, he got his first strike. He was so excited and proud of himself, that you could see the glow shinning off of his brow. Larry likes the white salamander so much that he never put another type of lure or color of lure on his pole again. To him it was no longer just a white salamander it was now "white death". Every time one of us would catch a fish we would laugh and yell white death strikes again.

I know I enjoyed the time fishing with Larry just as much if not more then he did. It was the start of me doing things that I used to do but now never found the time, energy, or the desire to do. It was so much more enjoyable to me then the new habits that I had picked up. It was one of the things that I needed to do to feel alive again. It was a great big step in the right direction of a better future for me, and was also the start of many fishing tales together.

I never told Larry how special our times were together or the fact that he was a part of me holding on to life. It seems like such a small thing to some, but to me it was a lot more. Thanks Larry you do deserve your own chapter in my book. I am always ready to set the hook with you again.

27

DIVORCE

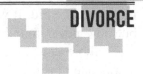

IT HAD TO HAPPEN SOONER or later because there was no way of changing my life if I had to deal with the same old wife and all her spending. I did get a kick out of the fact that she was the one who had me served with the divorce papers. I did go to a lawyer looking to file for a divorce a couple months before but did not want to pay them all the money they wanted to start the action, but after I got served I had no choice but to get a lawyer to protect myself.

It should have been a short cut and dry divorce, but then again nothing is ever that simple. Hell I could write a book just on the divorce alone. When the Opting Out Agreement was finally reached I felt like she had gotten the better end of things but my first concern was keeping my camp, so I was willing to give a little more. The biggest issue was our house which in the end we agreed would be sold and that she would get the assets from the sale. My concern now was that she would not sell it and we would be back in court a year later dealing with the same issues again. I was assured that this would not happen and that my name would be taken off the deed so I agreed.

Now since my credit was destroyed from bills not being paid when I was away she had to get a loan for me to get a car. Funny as it sounds because I co-signed for her all of my credit was shit and hers was great. Well when things started to go downhill between us I started to pay the car payment late every month. Oh I had the money but I waited on purpose and laughed about it to myself. It had to have affected her credit score some. So when she went to refinance she could not even though we only owed 20,000 on the house. Of course this made me smile. I wonder if she ever figured out that it was me that affected her credit score? LOL.

My x-wife was getting over 1,000 dollars a month from me in child support and maintenance payments. You would think that she would at least make the mortgage payments on time. Nope she got months behind which in the end ended up fucking both of us. I don't know what she did with her money; of course I never understood how someone could spend so much and have so little to show for it.

She took the house off the market the very next month after we signed the agreement, maybe in her defense it was because she wanted to refinance, but the agreement was to get the mortgage out of my name and when she could not refinance it she needed to sell it. Now when I called her on taking the house off the market she said that her lawyer said she did not have to sell it. Here we go right where I was afraid we would be. So I went back to my lawyer who wrote to her lawyer about what was going on. When nothing changed I had to take her back to court. The Court system sure moves slow and I tried to have patients with it, even though sometimes I thought it was against me.

My youngest moved in with me when we separated and we moved 30 miles away, but when I found out how hard of a time our middle child was having with everything, I moved back to that school district to get custody of her in the hopes that it would change her outlook on life. My x-wife's only concern was the amount of money she would lose in support. I laughed at her when I told her she would lose 600 dollars a months. She refused to pay me the child support that was owed to me according to our divorce agreement. Of course I stopped paying her the support but kept paying her the alimony checks even though it was more then she would be getting a month from me now. My lawyer told me to deduct the amount of child support she owes me from her alimony but I refused. I told him that I did not want there to be any area that I was in default when I finally got in front of the judge.

Not only was she not paying the mortgage payments but she also did not pay for 1200 dollars worth of propane that was delivered and the account was still in my name. It was in collection before I knew anything about it. Great another hit on my credit score. I called the collection agency who told me what was in default so I then went to the propane company and explained that I did not want to pay the bill until I got something in writing stating that she would repay me for the debt. Even though it stated that in the Opting Out Agreement I want something specific to each area she owed.

So again I go back to my lawyer and asked for her to pay anything she was in default for and also my lawyer fees, A clause she had her lawyer put in the Opting Out Agreement that the one in default would pay for the others lawyer. How stupid can one be to insure that and

RETIRED MSG DENNIS JAMES WILLIAMS

then default on any of the bills? Even funnier is when her lawyer wrote back and said not to send her anymore correspondence because she was not representing her anymore. Maybe she forgot to pay that bill also. LOL.

Now she goes to the court house and files a complaint, and I get served with papers for not paying child support. The court papers state that I need to bring everything about my finances to court and that I will be asked to answer these charges and that I could be arrested if I was found in default. So I make out a nice chart of all payments made, get copies of all checks she cashed and show up to court.

My first court appearance in front of the judge really rubbed me the wrong way. You could tell, or should I say it felt to me like the judge was favoring her side over mine. I sat there nice and quietly as she stated that I have not been paying child support payments and that she is responsible for her daughter and that until she gets something that says otherwise then she deserves the child support. Then the judge turns to me and asks me to explain things to him.

"I don't understand why I am here your honor? I have here in front of me a list of all payments made to her since the agreement was signed. I have paid her every payment on time up to September when Danielle moved in with me, and according to our agreement which has all the figures already done, I am entitled to so much a month since then. She has refused to pay me anything."

"Mrs. Williams did Danielle move in with Mr. Williams in September?" The judge asked.

"Yes but I am legally responsible for her and until I get something that states that I am not he needs to pay me the support."

"First of all you are responsible for your daughters no matter where they live as we have joint custody. Asking for a letter stating otherwise will never happen unless you give up your rights." I said to her.

The judge then says that "we will have to set a date to discuss this at a later date." And then asks his **secretary** what date he has available.

"I don't understand why we can't finish this today? I brought all the information you requested, and all the figures have already been agreed upon." I said

"I don't have the time to deal with this today." The judge said.

"Then what the hell did you tell me to come with everything then."

At this time I stood up and grabbed my papers and started to leave. The sheriff stopped me and gave me the paper with the next court date on it. I could hear the judge talking but I did not listen and continued on my way out. Hind sight I would have to say it was a stupid move and it could have gotten me in more trouble. The problem was that I was not thinking I was reacting. If only my lawyer made it to court. That is why I had one to keep me grounded so I don't get into trouble.

When we finally did get everyone into court together the judge took us into his chambers to see if there was anyway that we could settle this between ourselves so he would not have to rule.

"It would be in everyone's best interest if we could settle this." The judge said.

"Mrs. Williams has refused to except a full listed purchase price, she has refused to show the property to potential buyers, and took the house off the market one month after the Opting Out Agreement was signed." My lawyer stated.

"Mrs. Williams was you ever given a purchase price offer for the said resident? It does not matter if it was not a full offer under the circumstances you are obligated to accept any offer." The judge asked.

"That was not true I was never offered the full purchase price. The only offer that I got was for $35,000.00 by a family member of his, and the Opting Out Agreement states that I have a reasonable amount of time. My oldest child graduates in September and I want to stay there until then, and then I will move away to where she goes to college" My x-wife stated.

195

"Your honor we have the listing agent in the court room with proof that Mrs. Williams not only refused to accept any offer she also refused to show the residence." My lawyer stated.

"Mrs. Williams if are unable to refinance the mortgage on said property then you have no choice but to sell it, and it does not have to be the full purchase price. Waiting till September is not reasonable. I suggest that you and Mr. Williams go to the office upstairs and try to come to sort of agreement that must be followed in order to put these matters behind us." The judge said.

We all agreed to try one last time and my lawyer, my x-wife, the realtor, and I went to the room and sat down to draw up a binding contract that would be followed. I told my lawyer that I wanted her thrown out of the house and that I would make the payments until it was sold, and that if she was out I would be able to make any repairs necessary. He told me the judge would never go for that and that we could take her out of the equation about what amount would be accepted by having it approved by both you and the realtor. My x-wife tried to find a way so she could still keep the property and my lawyer told her we were way beyond that point now.

In the end it was agreed upon that the records would show that I had physical custody of both younger children and that the alimony would be offset by the child support. It was also agreed upon that the realtor would make the decision on what was or was not a reasonable offer and that both parties agreed that the realtor's opinion and Mr. William's opinion would be the only two who had to agree to the sale. Mrs. Williams would repay Mr. Williams for the propane, back child support, back mortgage payment, his lawyer and any amount paid to the mortgage over what her allotted amount for the month would be.

We all went back in front of the judge with our agreement and he asked all parties if they agreed with the stipulation and if they were satisfied. When the judge asked me I told him I was willing to accept the terms but that I did not agree with them. Of course the judge asked me further question so that he felt that I understood what was being agreed upon. He then stated that if both parties feel they are unhappy with the decision then maybe it is a better decision. The judge agreed to accept the agreement and it was so sworn in.

We started the house on the market at $49,900.00 just like last time. After a couple months I request to have it lowered and the realtor agreed. We were a little concerned that my x would not agree to this but she signed the papers without any questions. We lowered it to $45,000 and still no offers. Of course the fact that there was a busted pipe that destroyed the kitchen floor and by the time she got the pipe fixed the floor was all warped and soft. Now the insurance would have paid for it to get fixed if only she was that smart. I surely did not say anything. The cheaper it was sold the less she would get. LOL. Maybe you think this is cruel and wrong of me to not say anything but to me it was like waking up to a bright sunny day. Of course the down side was that it was harder to get the place approved for a mortgage loan from a bank, but in the end it did not matter because it went for $32,000.00 and the guy paid cash. Hell I think he stole the place.

I wish I could say that was the end of the drama but it was not. I do not know how someone could act the way that my x-wife did. In the end she hurt herself more then she did me. She should have walked away with almost $30,000.00 but in the end I don't think she even got $6,000.00. Seems she was in default on the credit cards that she was supposed to pay during the first agreement and they put a lien on the house until it was paid. It cost me having to wait longer to buy my next house because she had me as an authorized user. How can that be on my credit report against me is a mystery. I was in the attempt of getting a house loan through the VA, and you can't be late on anything for a year. I got the loan company to overlook the mortgage, but when the credit card popped up it was the end of my quest for buying a new home at this time.

I smile whenever I think of how she screwed herself out of so much money, but in the end the ones that she hurt the most is our two youngest daughters that are now living with me. Their mother has refuse to see them or talk to them and even refused to see them last Christmas. I try and I try to get the kids and even her to reach out to the other but it is all in vain. I wonder if she knows how much pain she is causing them? I try and deal with their issue, and I wish I could say I was doing a great job but I do not think that I am. How can I even think of a way to make them understand that their mother refuses to see them yet has all the time in the world for their older sister? I hated telling them that their mother did not want them for Christmas, but I did cherish the emotional moment with my middle child. She let me hold her tight as she cried in my arms. All I could do was tell her I was sorry and that I loved her, but still I don't think it eased the pain that her mother had caused.

Now I count the number of payments that I have to make to her before the tide turns and she has to pay me. I offered to just wipe the slate clean before she had to pay me but she wanted me to pay. She is a fool because in the end it is going to cost her because she is going to pay me more then I had to pay her. LOL. Other then that everyday I know that she is farther out of my life then the day before. Like a cancer that is being fought. It did not kill me and I am starting to see a change in the fight. Can't wait for the doctor to say I am cancer free.

28

TRIPS

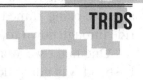

EVEN THOUGH I WAS STILL married my relationship with my new girl friend was moving forward. We had lots of issues that we needed to iron out, and I can say that it took a lot of work on both our parts, but in the end we always seem to come back together. Is that not what building a relationship is, the give and take that you both make to bond yourselves to one another? Well we had lots of bonding, and I can say that a lot of it was because I was still on my way of changing things and I still went back and forth from the old life to the new one I was trying to make.

There was / are many aspects of her that drew me to her. The physical attraction was there, and the fact that she needed someone as much as I needed someone sure helped. The more I learned about her and her desires the more I long to live again and to do those things that inspired her and my soul so long ago. She never has been anywhere really and she so wanted to experience everything in life. Some people say this and they are mainly just talking shit, but I can tell you this she meant everything she said.

Our trips started out as day trips where we would drive there, spend the day, and then drive back home. We went on a trip to Niagara Falls and the jet boats up to the whirl pool. I had done it before so I made sure we got there first to get a front seat. It was a wet wild ride just like I remembered. At one point I thought I had pressure washed my brain with the amount of water that engulfed us. I saw the look of fear in her eye, even if she contests that it was not fear but surprise.

We had a few day trips down to New York City. The Bronx Zoo is a great day trip because it does not open until 10 o'clock, so if you leave around six a.m. you will get there just as it opens. You spend the day there then stop in Newburgh for dinner and then the ride home. We also stopped at South Pier, and took the free bus to Battery Park, and then to the Empire State building. I don't mind visiting the city but I surely don't want to live there.

We went to Boston Massachusetts three different times, once to Salem and twice to the Aquarium. I enjoyed the aquarium much more then I did Salem and the museums of the witches. We even got to view a movie being filmed in Boston as we were taking a horse and buggy ride through down town.

One night we were home and talking and she mentioned that her husband was going down south and that he was going to see a Dallas Cowboys game in Dallas. I said to her don't be jealous if you want to go there we will. I don't think she believed me by her comment, but I just got on the internet and looked and the schedule for the Cowboys and our work schedule and found the most feasible game and bought two tickets, and then made flight and hotel arrangements for a week there. We had a great time in Texas; we went horse back riding for two hours, made it to a rodeo in Fort Worth Stockyards, and went to Medieval Times, the Fort Worth Zoo, Ripley's Believe It Or Not wax Museum, as well as got to watch the Philadelphia Eagles beat the Dallas Cowboys in their new stadium. Funniest story was when we kept driving in circles looking for the stadium that you think would be easy to find. After all it is kind of big. Finally we saw a guy on the side of the road so we asked him where it was.

He laughed and said "you are standing on it now, but they built a new one."

"I guess that would explain why we could not find it."

We did get a good chuckle out of it. I even offered to pick up a stone that used to be the stadium. Sounds funny now but you should have been there with us trying to understand what was going on and her trying to read the GPS as I was driving trying to follow her directions.

We talked about our next vacation and where we should go. We both wanted Las Vegas so I made the arrangements. I was told that you should make all your plans in advance for the shows to make sure they are not sold out so we sat down and figured out what we wanted to do. It was a fun adventure filled week and I know we both would love to go back again. There is so much to do and so much to see. Here is what we did.

1) We went to Boot Mountain and did the zip line, which I highly recommend, hell the bus ride up was as much excitement with the steep cliffs and narrow roads as the ride down was. Being

in the bus if you looked out the window you could not see the dirt roads under you. The zip line was a series of platforms that took you down the mountain at speeds of 50 mph. it was worth every penny and I highly recommend it. Ever imagined what it'd be like to soar from the top of a mountain with an eagle's eye view? Or envisioned a new eco-friendly way to explore mountain terrain without leaving a trace of your journey behind? Then let your imagination become reality and experience the thrill and the beauty of Boulder City's newest eco-adventure at the base of Red Mountain—the Bootleg Canyon Zip line Tour. Suspended from cables and comfortably sitting in a Para-gliding harness, you travel from point to point by flying over the desert ecosystem from the top of Red Mountain.

2) We drove to the Grand Canyon and along the way we stopped many times to take pictures and look at the breath taking view around us. We ended up at The Hualapai Nation of The Grand Canyon West, where you had to take a bus to get any closer. I could not believe it, there was no fences no guide wires, nothing to stop you from falling over the side. What a view and what a walk. They have a Sky Walk there where you are walking on glass looking straight down to the bottom of the canyon. Believe me it is a weird feeling. It was even funny watching the young lady who was laughing at the way some of the people were acting scared out on the walk, and when it was her turn she lost control of her self and started crying. It was funny watching them carry her off. I had so much fun there that I had to take a souvenir, so I acquired a nice size rock from one of the fire places in an Indian teepee. Shame on me LOL. I also got to see a wild Pronghorn sheep, which might not be much for the locals, but to me it was exciting.

3) On the way back from the Grand Canyon we stopped at the Hoover Dam. Wow is all I can say. How could something so big be built so long ago, and if that is not enough the bridge for the high way that goes over the dam is just as impressive. I had to call my mother from the bridge and say to her look I am

traveling in time, as I jumped from one time zone to the next. Of course she did not understand what I was saying or doing so I had to explain it to her. LOL. On the way out of the dam I got to see a herd of Big Horn Sheep and watch a big Ram jump across the road right in front of us and climb the mountain side. How the hell do they do that without falling? Again to some they are just an everyday sight but to me it was magical.

4) We did some gambling. People must have thought we were winning a lot of money the way we hollered over winning a quarter or two. I think we only spent about 50 dollars in all gambling the entire week we was there and we won most of that back. Casinos did not make much on us.

5) We went on the Price is Right show at Bally's. We never got called to contestant row but we paid the extra to be right in front of the stage. Of course they made it interesting by having everything priced from back in the 70's. They called new people up for every bid and gave those that did not make it to the stage a tee-shirt.

6) Rod Stewart at the Colosseum was one of the shows that we saw. The funniest thing was that the casino said that no pictures could be taken and the first thing Rod did was to tell everyone that he did not care what the casino said and that you could take all the pictures and videos that you wanted. It was an amazing show where he sang and took the time to make everyone in the arena feel like they were a part of the show. He even showed pictures of his family and talked about them. Then he started kicking soccer balls out into the crowd and every one went crazy. It was one of my favorite concerts that I have ever gone to.

7) Terry Fator at the Mirage was the third show that we went to. I did not really know who he was but she said he was funnier then hell and that he did puppets and sang. I have to say it was hilarious. The different characters and voices that he used just kept you on the edge of your feet. Then he asked for a

volunteer from the crowd and he got even funnier. He had the guy stand there and put an outfit on him where he controlled the mouth of the mask. He added a yellow long hair wig and spoke as a woman. The man seemed like a natural and moved his arms as if he was talking and posing as a girl. I can still see the sight in my mind. He gave the guy some signed pictures of the two of them as well as a shirt. A once in a life time thrill.

8) We stayed at the Stratosphere Casino. Of course she wanted to do the sky jump, which is the ultimate Vegas free fall from the 108th floor where blood curdling screams can be heard in the sky high above the Las Vegas Strip. Stratosphere's new Sky Jump thrill ride is not for the faint of heart, and will be the jump of your life. It must have been made for those adrenaline junkies wanting the ultimate free fall, without going out of a plane. It provides the highest controlled free fall in the world, all from the Stratosphere Tower. Believe it or not I have jumped from airplanes in the service much lower then this altitude. Before the jump, we were prepped and suited up in Stratosphere's custom jump suits and given our safety briefing. I mean what can they say don't mess your pants on the way down because someone is under you? Then you are taken up to the jumping platform and connected to their high-speed "descended" and led to the edge of the platform where you take that last step and plummet through the sky 855 feet, or the equivalent of 108 floors. We watched the people before us and I had to smile at the way most of them timidly fell off the platform. Of course she had to go before me. She did not hesitate to step off the platform and down she went. Next was my turn and after I got to the ledge I check everything as if I was standing in the door of a C-130 and then jumped as far out as I could. Of course there was no tight body position; I was more like superman flying through the air with my arms and legs stretched out as far as I could. It was just what it said it was a freefall to the ground where the stop was a quick little jerk. The downside is that the freefall is not that long and before you know it is all over.

9) Also on the top of the Stratosphere there are three rides. I did not want to do them but she made me. LOL. She even made me do them at night just so it would be that much more of a thrill.

- The first one we did was the Big Shot which shot you160 feet in the air at 45 miles per hour. As if you were not high enough as it was. In a matter of seconds, the Big Shot thrill ride catapults 16 riders from the 921-foot high platform up the Tower's mast to a height of 1,081 feet and down again. Before you catch your breath, you'll be shot back up again. We experience a gut-wrenching four 'G's of force on the way up, and felt the negative 'G's on the way down as our legs dangle in the Las Vegas skyline. This was a nice ride that made a breath taking view of the city even better. The lady running the ride said most people save this ride for last and I said nope this is our first because when we do the one that goes in a circle I will be done.

- The second ride was called the X-Scream and was 866 feet above the ground. The X-Scream resembles a massive teeter-totter or a Vegas rollercoaster unlike any other ever seen. X-Scream propels you and several other riders headfirst, 27 feet over the edge of the Stratosphere Tower. After being shot over the edge, you'll dangle weightlessly above the Las Vegas Strip before being pulled back and propelled over again for more. It looked pretty scary from the side lines and of course as fait would have it we ended up in the front seat. The track rose up and the car shot down the 27 feet over the edge to stop suddenly and then lift up and down. We both laughed our asses off on this one. It went back and forth a couple times and then was done.

- The last ride was the Insanity and it was the one that I dreaded. This thrill ride is 3 'G's of pure Insanity and is a truly mind-bending experience. A massive mechanical arm extending out 64 feet over the edge of the Stratosphere Tower at a height of over 900 feet, this Vegas ride will spin you and several other passengers in the open air at speeds of up to three 'G's. You'll be propelled up to an angle of 70 degrees, which will tilt your body into one position—straight down! If you're brave enough to keep your eyes open you'll be rewarded with a breathtaking view of historic downtown Las Vegas. The height did not bother me but once it started I knew I was in trouble. I tried to keep my composure but the turning and the bright lights made me dizzy and I felt light headed and I wanted to puke. The fact that she sat there next to me trying to keep me calm the entire time just made things worse. When I got off the ride I felt weak and faint, and I knew I was done for the night. Of course she just laughed at me.

10) Another thing she had never done that she wanted to do was to ride in a helicopter. We did not have the time for the all day trip but I called to go on the Maverick Night Flight across the strip. When you got there they gave you a shirt and a glass of champagne. There were three couples in our group on the bird and when we got to it the pilot asked if one of the couples did not mind splitting up so we all could get a better view because the strip is on the same side going each way. Since I have been on many helicopters in my days I volunteered to be split up from her as long as she got the best seat. The pilot agreed and put her in the co-pilot's seat. It was a nice 20 minute ride where you taxied out over the runway for a good distance just off the ground before you took off. I did not think there was a bad seat in the bird because it was almost all windows, though I could tell she was enjoying the co-pilot's seat. When the flight was over she told me she was so tempted to grab a hold of the throttle and fly the bird. I just laughed. What an adrenaline junkie I got here.

11) There is two aquariums in Las Vegas one is full of sharks and the other one full of dolphins. She wanted to go see the dolphins because she never saw a real one before. I agreed only if she would go to the shark one. She is deathly afraid of sharks and I had to use my great knowledgeable brain so I would be able to see the sharks. We did have fun in both though, and they did not take long so we fit them in around our other scheduled shows.

Las Vegas sure is full of things to do and see. Even the times that we spent walking down the strip gave us something to talk about. From the people with the signs asking for money for all different reasons from a breast enlargement, money for a drink, to a guy stating you could kick him in the balls for 10 dollars. Then you got the people at every street crossing trying to give you the pamphlets of the hot girls to your room within 20 minutes. They were everywhere, funny how they hit the pamphlet on there hand before trying to pass them out. If you think that was openly asking for you to get a girl you should see the trucks with the billboards on them just driving around with those hot almost naked women on them with the number to call. Then you had all those people in costumes of just about any cartoon charter you could think of, hoping you would take a picture with them for tips. The ones I wanted to take my picture with I did not dare because she was there. How can those girls be on the street with what they were wearing! Would have been a sin in other cities. Sin city I can see why it got that name, where ever you go or look it is there in front of you, and it's all legal.

12) I would have to say the biggest thrill for both of us was the one that I surprised her with. After all the plans had been made I made reservations for tandem sky diving. She had been telling me since I have been talking to her about how much she wanted to go. I did take her parasailing twice but if you ever jumped from a plane and then went parasailing you would see how boring parasailing really is. I mean there is no depth perception because you are over water and there is no thrill of leaving the plane. The scheduled day came and we went through the ten minute film and signed the wavers. We got all suited up and then the jump was canceled because of the wind. The next chance we got to go they wanted us there early to go before their scheduled jumps. It was a good thing because we were the only flight to get off that day. We got there suited us up and off we went to the plane.

"Are you scared or nervous?" My flight buddy asked me.

"Let me see, I did the sky jump yesterday, I have done the indoor free falling towers twice, and I was an airborne ranger. Nope I don't think I am that scared or nervous." I said.

"I was 5th special forces out of Fort Bragg." He said.

"Hell we walked across the same sand path." I said.

"You are going to go off first."

"Don't you want to go over hooking up with me?" I said

"Nope we will do it in the plane." My jump buddy said.

I knew she wanted to jump out of the plane before, but I did not say anything about that to him. We had to wait for all the others to load the plane and then we sat down by the door. It was a small plane where the three buddy teams of jumpers filled the entire plane. It was a short flight but I did enjoy it, even though the noise and feel of the harness brought back memories of my younger days. I was instructed to grab a bar and pull myself up so he could snap my harness to his. Then he opened the door and we slid around to where my feet were hanging out the door. Hell I was almost all the way out just sitting in the breeze at 15,000 feet.

Next thing I knew I was falling as if in a dream. I saw my shoes and the ground below me, then the sky, the plane, and then the ground again. I was a little surprised that it looked just like any normal jump. I mean the summersault that the body goes through before it gets stable. I held on to my harness like I was instructed and grinned from ear to ear. Forgetting all about the instruction to hold my arms straight out after we get out. I was so lost in my own excitement that he had to hit me a few times before I realized that he wanted me to open my arms to help keep us stable. I opened my arms and we each gave the other thumbs up.

There is no possible way that I can correctly describe the feeling that I was feeling as I was falling at 120mph for 45 seconds. We were so high that I felt a temperature change as we were descending. I can still see the view and feel as if I am now out there falling and smiling and looking around trying to take everything in. The 45 seconds seemed like an eternity of heavenly bliss. I could not believe how long we fell before he finally pulled the ripcord to deploy the chute.

I remember how surprised I was with the quick slight jerk that I felt as the wind filled the chute. It was nothing like the feeling that I have felt from those military chutes when they snap you back. I remember saying shit to myself and feeling let down as we stopped falling and came to a nice floating state. I looked around and asked where the others were, and smiled when he pointed her out to me. I know she must be in heaven right now in her mind.

"Are you ready Joe?"

"Sure you got the reins." I said.

In hind sight I should have told him that I was just fine with a slow descent. They did tell us in the beginning that the chute would open at 5,000 feet and from there you could chose between a slow and a faster more energetic descent. Maybe because he knew I was an Airborne Ranger in my youth that I was ready for anything because all of a sudden I was being zipped around in a circle one way and then the other. At first I was surprised and enjoyed the thrill, but I soon became a little dizzy and nauseated. I did not have it in me to tell him to stop so around and around we went all the way to the ground where he told me to land flat on my butt. Sounds funny but if you jumped all the time with people strapped to you that you did not know it would be a lot safer then trying to have them land on their feet and stay standing. Swoosh we slide on the nice hot Nevada sand.

As soon as I get unhooked I bent over to throw up but nothing came but air. Good thing I did not eat breakfast. I sure felt like crap and again the feeling of throwing up came to me and I sprinted to the edge of their little DZ. Again I tried to empty my stomach but there was nothing in there. I stayed there bent over until I finally felt clear headed and then went over to her and asked her how it was. She just looked at me with a glow in her eyes and said she did not know how to explain what she had just experienced. I just smiled and said "you don't have to."

13) It was a long and exhausting week. Finally Saturday came and we were laying in bed at 600am when I rolled over and asked her to marry me today. It was not planned it just seem like the thing to do. We got up and went to breakfast and then set out to find a couple rings for us. After we got the rings we went to the court house to apply for a marriage licenses. There was the same gauntlet of people with advertisements as on the strip. The only difference was that here they were trying to get you to go to their chapel. When we got inside the court house is was like a DMV office with twelve rows of windows to apply for marriage licensees, and there was the rope in area to wait for the next available teller. Of course there was a waiting line as well. LOL.

After we got our licenses we drove to A Little White Wedding Chapel. Yes it is the one from Hangover and Friends. She is a Friend fans so it just seems like the perfect place to go. As we got there we could see that it was crowded so we kept on driving. We stopped at the first parking lot we saw and I called them looking to get an appointment time. The lady said don't worry about the people here we got lots of people who can marry you. When would you like to get married? I looked at the time and it was 1255pm, and I told her we wanted to get married at 1305pm. I thought maybe I would catch her off guard but I did not and she said to come on down. We got there and signed in, and we were asked what kind of wedding we wanted. They offered a drive through service, Elvis, inside a pink Cadillac, and religion, hell I think they did just about anything anyone wanted to have the perfect wedding. We just wanted something simple in the chapel. As I looked around I saw that they had every last minute thing that one would want at a wedding. I grabbed a nice set of flowers and she smiled when I gave them to her.

We needed a witness so we got this old lady who played the organ to be our witness. We were a mess; she had on flip flops because of the blisters on her feet from her new shoes that she had to wear walking everywhere. There would be no walking down the aisle here, we stood side by side and said our vows. We paid for two songs on the organ but I did not hear any music. I was so caught up in the moment. After we went outside and had some pictures taken and then off we went as man and wife.

Both of us agree that it was the best week of our lives, fun exciting, full of challenge, and with the perfect ending. We could not have planned a better wedding if we tried. Maybe it was not as glamorous of a wedding as most people try for but it was more personal and emotional then anyone could plan. Together she and I have been taking on the world for the last couple of years. A lot of ups and also a lot of downs, but there we were on the spur of the moment standing at the alter hand and hand pledging to be not just man and wife but life long partners and friends till then end. Hell Harry and Sally could not have done it better.

29

HEAVY HEART

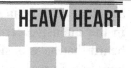

IT COMES WITH A HEAVY heart that I add this chapter to my book. They say that there is good in anything, and I guess it is true though sometimes the good is not really wanted but accepted because there is no other choice. In my struggles to find myself and a reason to make it to tomorrow or to find some kind of spark of feelings inside of myself, I have done many things as you have read. Some of these things could be considered good or bad depending on your outlook of things. I have done drugs and alcohol to sooth the feeling of nothingness that was growing inside of me; I tried to live through others. In the end I made the decision to live, to find a way to overcome the feelings of aloneness or the feelings of not fitting in or wanting to fit in.

I have to say that I have come along way; even so my therapist tells me that I should feel sad about something. Maybe even cry some tears. It just was never there. I had lots of other feeling but to really be sad about anything just never really hit home to me. It seems like such a stupid thing to be able to cry. I mean men don't cry right. Men are big and strong they are like rocks, real men anyways. The tears have not flowed down my cheeks but I feel them in my eyes. My eyes feel so full of sorrow that it wants to just break down and bawl like a baby.

The service tends to make one cold. How else can you deal with the aspects of war, of seeing the death and destruction that comes with it? How else can you go on when the one that you have depended on for everything is hurt or gone in front of your eyes? You can not just turn a switch and become human again. It is instilled inside of your brain, inside of the core of ones sole.

My family has always complained about me being cold when it came to people dying. I never go up to see the body and I never show any kind of feelings toward them. Usually I would just make a smart ass comment like there is more room in the world, or there is another job opening. Sounds cruel I do agree. I must have looked like a cruel person to them. They must have thought how I could be so cold or rude.

Recently a fellow co-worker passed away. He was not killed in an accident or anything sudden like that. He got sick and spent a month in the intensive care unit in the hospital. I was shocked when I first heard that he was sick in the hospital. My first thought when I heard how bad he was, was that he would not make it but I so did not want this that I hung on to any little change, any little hope that he would get better. I read his and his wife's face book pages at least twice a day hoping to see some good news. His wife always sounded positive in his recovery that I began to believe it. In the end it was not to be and he passed away.

This was not just another co-worker. This was Vlad! This was a man who spoke his mind, who carried himself with pride, and who did not believe an apple was an orange just because someone else said it was. People always joked about his conspiracy theory. I never joked about them, I listened to his reasoning and we spoke of most everything, from politics, weapon control, fluoride in our drinking water, to making cookies.

We always spoke every time we saw each other. If he did not come up to me I was sure to come up to him and shake his hand, slap his gut or give him a big hug. We had our little unspoken game of who could find and wear the most absurd shirt to work. He had a lot of great ones, the one I liked the most was the one that had a guy on suicide watch eating popcorn as you saw behind him the man he was expose to be watching hanging by a rope. Surely it could not be a proper shirt to wear in a place where we work. I finally thought I had him when I got this pink shirt that said "Don't laugh it is your girlfriend's shirt" on it.

Vlad always spoke his mind to me as I did to him. I am sure that we both shared the same respect for each other, and I also am sure that no matter what the situation was that we had each others back. He was so full of life and always spoke of his son, and his dogs. He always cheered me up when I was having a difficult time at work. He asked for nothing in return but for me to just be me. He gave me lots of his wisdom, and I can honestly say that he showed me that there was a reason to live. He made me feel good about the things that I have done in my life.

Since I heard the bad news that he passed away I have been emotionally destroyed. I see him in my mind all day long. Work seems so quiet it is almost surreal. I keep waiting for him to come to work and brighten the place up. He had a way with his laughter, and his love for life, to make everyone feel alive. Everyone loved him, well I loved him and it seemed like he got along with everyone.

Vlad's wife asked for everyone to wear green to show support for him. Some say I went a little overboard, but I don't think I did enough to show what he meant to me. My wife and I spent an entire day shopping for things to wear to his calling hours, and his funeral. My wife even said I did not have to go to such extreme, but I was set in my mind to do as Vlad would expect me to do. I bought new green shoes, and greenish socks. I say greenish socks because one might say they were more yellow then green but it was as close to green that I could get. I also got green shorts and three green shirts. One was a regular pullover shirt that was green and on it in big letters was "SMOKE POT, and PLAY VIDEO GAMES," which was Vlad to a tee. I also bought a green shirt that had a picture on it so it looked like it was a suit. It had a bow tie and Irish buttons on it. The last was a green button up shirt, which was a little dressy. Then I got some green hair dye, and some green nail polish.

The night before his wake I dyed my hair and colored my finger nails. To me there was not that much green in my hair but my wife said you could see it. That's what happens when you have dark hair and you color it without bleaching it first. I also printed a picture of Vlad and placed it over my picture on my work badge. A lot of people put pictures on their badges of people as a joke; I did it out of respect for him. I wore my green shoes, socks, shorts, and put on the shirt that said "SMOKE POT and PLAY VIDEO GAMES." I knew that this shirt was pushing the line at work so I brought the other green pull over incase I was told I had to change my shirt. I did make it through the entire day with the shirt on. Of course I got comments from most people both patients and staff.

I was lucky enough to get out of work on time and I went and picked up my wife and we went to the funeral parlor. I had with me in a plastic bag a flag that I bought the day before that I had folded into the shape of a paper football, and the Army Accommodation medal that I received in Iraq. The line was long when we got there; in the end the line was long for six hours as people came to pay their respects to him. As my wife and I got to the casket I climbed up and placed the flag inside next to him, and then pinned the medal on his chest. I then just stood there a minute rubbing his arm up and down. A lot of memories were running through my head about him. I did not want to walk away because I did not want it to be true.

Finally my wife was able to pull me from the casket we stopped and paid out respects to his family standing there. I noticed that his wife was not there at this time so I asked where she was and was told that her family made her take a break. I saw where she was sitting down and went over to her and gave her a hug. I told her that I was sorry that things ended this way and that I put a flag in his casket and a medal on his chest. I told her he was the truest American that I ever knew. She told me she loved the shirt that I was wearing and that Vlad would have liked it. I smiled as good of a smile as I could muster to her and said "I know," and then left.

It was a very emotional time for me, almost more then I could handle, and even though I was glad to be out of the funeral home I was still sadden by the turn of events that got me there in the first place. My wife and I spoke about the time spent inside over dinner. She could tell that Vlad was special to me and that I was taking it hard.

The next morning was the funeral services and then to the cemetery. I wore the same shorts, socks, and shoes but put the other two shirts on. I made sure we got there early because I wanted to get a good seat. The funeral parlor filled up fast and they brought in extra chairs. The music was typical funeral music maybe just a little lower volume then normal. All of a sudden the music started blaring out of the speakers, and everyone laughed. Seemed Vlad was going out with a lot of thunder just like he lived, and the music was not one of a funeral but one of life being lived to the fullest.

Then the preacher that was from the hospital started the ceremony. He spoke how he never saw so many people so concerned over any patient before. Seemed all the hospitals employees were talking about Vlad and how his progress was going. I know it could have not been from Vlad's charm that got them so interested. I have to believe that it was the love and caring and devotion that not only his wife and family showed but also his co-workers. He also led everyone in prayer and read from the bible and spoke of meeting Vlad again.

Vlad's mother spoke next, and I have to say that it tore my heart apart to listen to her speak of her son. It was such and emotional moment, you could tell that they had a special bound between them. She had a tough time and had to stop a couple times to keep a hold of herself. She walked over to the casket and spoke to him. It was a beautiful moment in my eyes and I am sure it will last in her mind forever also.

Next a friend of the family spoke. I did not catch much of what she said, not to say that it was not emotional or anything. It was just that I was so caught up in Vlad's mother speech that I did not follow the next speaker. When she got done the preacher asked if anyone else had anything to say.

I could not sit there and not say something out of respect for Vlad, I knew if I did not it would bother me the rest of my life so I stood and said I would like to say something. I don't know if I sounded as unsettled as it sounded to me but I know I was struggling to hold on to my composure. I started off talking about how Vlad and I would always say hello when we saw each other at work. If not a hand shake or a punch in the gut it would be a hug. Vlad and I were like women always comparing what we were wearing to each others and trying to get the most comical shirt saying. Vlad told me he ordered his shirts on line and that I should take a look at this site, though I never did. I know I got him when I wore the pink shirt to work that said "DON'T LAUGH, IT'S YOUR GIRLFRIEND SHIRT." I always got a lot of laughs over that one and Vlad laughed his ass off over it. Still the shirt that he wore with a guy eating popcorn with a person hanging themselves behind them with the saying "SUCIDE WATCH," was always my favorite even though I never told him that. I spoke of how Vlad was always there to give me some strength when I needed it and that he would have expected me to speak on his behalf.

Vlad always had this big "CONSPIRACY" theory about the government, and his favorite saying was that "PROUD TO BE AMERICAN—ASHAMED OF MY GOVERNMENT. I spoke that Vlad was the most dedicated American that I knew because of his theories, and that if everyone followed our leaders blindly we would be a dictatorship instead of a democratic country. I stated that Vlad was my friend and that "I had no problem at all saying I loved him and that I would miss him very much."

At this point I sat down and bawled like a baby. I could not stop and I did not care who saw me crying. After the ceremony many people came up to me and gave me a hug and told me that I did a wonderful job and showing how I felt about him. I was also yelled at by a couple because they had to fight to hold it together when his mother spoke but they could not after I spoke and that there was not a dry eye in the place. I did not notice any of that as I was still trying to get a hold of myself. I do know that I could have stood and talked a lot more if I could have just kept a hold of myself. Deep down I know that no matter what I said I could not express the amount of sadness that I felt at losing him.

After the ceremony my wife and I followed in the motorcade to the cemetery. Bag pipes were playing as the casket was brought out of the funeral parlor and at the cemetery. The preacher spoke again and then they passed out envelopes to people who opened them up and threw butterflies over the casket. It was such a tender moment. Vlad's wife brought his dog and wore Vlad's favorite sweatshirt. She cradled over the casket for a very long time, no an extremely long time. When she finally got off the casket people started going up to the casket to pay their last respects by either kissing or touching the casket. My wife tried to get me to go up but I refused to. I just stood there by myself in my own thoughts. I can still picture myself standing there now. My wife came back over to me and with the help of someone else and they got me to go see the casket. It was beautiful with his name and dates and a shamrock engraved into the wood. I am sure he would have been pleased himself at the quality of the casket.

After the cemetery they had a small gathering at his house. My wife and I went. We stayed a couple hours and had a few drinks and some food as we all spoke of our memories of Vlad. We had to leave early to get our kids so I gave Vlad's wife a hug goodbye and spoke of adding him to my book. She told me she knew he would love it and that she had no problem with it at all.

I later spoke to my therapist on the passing of my great friend and that I finally showed some emotions and cried. She always told me I needed to let myself be sad now and then and that it was not healthy to never be sad. Sad is not the word because I still think of him everyday and my eyes still water up, sometimes the tears just flow. It is hard to listen to others at work talk about him and not tear up. I have started answering line up like Vlad did, because it makes me feel like he is still there with us. He is still with me.

I chose to add this chapter out of respect for Vlad. Everyone always asked if they were in the book, and my answer was you don't want to be in the book because everyone in the book was no longer with us. I know Vlad was looking forward to reading it. Maybe most people would think that I am ending my book in a negative way? I guess it would fall down to your opinion on things. Vlad's passing was a terrible thing and I still wish it was not so, but it also showed me that I have come along way and that I cherish my life and look forward to tomorrow. Vlad was a wonderful friend, father, husband, and son and it made me realize that life is short and that we should make the most out of everyday we have.

To you my friend I say farewell, you were a true friend to me and I miss you a lot.

May the road rise up to meet you
May the wind be always at your back
May the sun shine warm upon your face
The rains fall soft upon your fields
And until we meet again
May God hold you in the palm of his hand

30

LOOKING FORWARD

I KNOW THAT I HAVE to remember what I have been through and how hard it was for me to make it to the point where I am. With the help from a therapist, and a psychiatrist along with some properly adjusted medication, I have found that living can be fun and that you can manage things in your past so that they don't destroy everything. It is hard, but then again anything worth wild is not easy. I try to be open and honest to my new wife and it feels good to be able to do this although there are still some things I don't share with her. My wife's desire to do new things and go to new places has inspired me to look past my kids growing up and look toward growing old with someone by my side. I am not saying that it is an easy thing to do, because it is not. We fight, and we don't understand each other at times but we try to. We try to be as much as a single unit as we can without taking away our souls. Although at times I still feel the urge to be alone somewhere by myself. I have to fight against myself so I don't get lost in this mental state. Like that addict I have to stay away from that first glass, that first puff, or first snort of cocaine, knowing that I still could slip back into myself. I truly understand how some veterans go off to the back woods somewhere and live their lives in harmony with themselves. I can see myself doing this very thing.

I still struggle at work, but I know that it is not that I can't handle any situation; rather I struggle with my work ethics and my integrity. The National Guard had a saying "Lead, Follow, or Get Out Of The Way." I attempted to be a leader and was shot down by management at work for what ever reason they had. I can't follow someone who does not lead even if they tell you they are leading. So I have chosen to get out of the way, and to stay as far away from any kind of decision at work. Of course that is unrealistic but I try none the less. I have to remind myself time and again that it is just a job and not a career.

The ties to my x-wife get shorter and shorter with each passing day. Her negative influence on my life steadily diminishes. Knowing that she hurt herself more then she has me makes it a little easier to live with, but does nothing to help me understand how or why she is as she is. I hate the fact that she does not see her two younger daughters but I also know that I have done just about everything I can think of to foster any kind of interaction between them.

My new wife and I talk about everything together. Even though we don't agree on some things we always find a happy medium or she always gets her way. LOL. We are looking forward to buying our own home and going places and doing things together. We deal with our issues as they come, even if she does not understand a lot of my lonely feelings or of my nightmares she makes me focus in the right direction.

I now know that the VA is a great help to me currently and will always be there in my future. I don't think of me as a war hero or even a hero. I did what I had to do when I had to do and did not question what I did. When I do think back about things that I did and choices that I made I know that if someone has not been in a situation like that they would question some of the orders and choices that I made and followed.

Everyone has there own ghost in the closet, and I am no exception to the rule. I don't really know what really took me over the edge. Was it the combat, and the blood and gore, was it dealing with the x-wife and the money when I got home, or was it work making me feel belittled. It most likely is a little of all three. I knew things were bothering me about what happened in Iraq even before I got back to the states. I did think about talking to someone during out-processing, but it went so fast I had no chance to really address anything. Then to deal with the money issue with someone who did not care about anything but herself. So I threw myself into worked and did what I thought was right and attempted to fix the issues and keep my family together. When I did finally get the chance to relax I noticed some of the bad habits that I had. Maybe management at work had their concerns about whether or not I could have handled anymore stress in my life, but them not helping me especially after I openly sought assistance is unforgivable.

I never asked to be put on a pedestal, and I never asked for any special favors. I openly sought out the reason for others decisions that they made and because I stood my ground and said "what the fuck" I was looked at as a trouble maker. I was someone who did not go with the flow. It did not matter that the flow was unjust. How I made it to the point I am today without pulling that trigger surely is a mystery in my mind. I know my kids stopped me a lot of times, but I think that work pissed me off, and belittled me so much that I made it my goal to seek out justice for myself.

There is no way that any amount of money for a settlement that will give me back what was taken from me. No money will ever change my opinion of what and who did what they did at work. Nothing my x-wife could do to change what she did to me and to my kids and our family. The past is the past and I have found a way to accept that. It was a long road with me questioning almost every decision that I made when I made one.

I have no remorse for following someone else's wishes for so long. I have no remorse about going through the cycle that I did with the alcohol, drugs and running around. I did what I did to make it through to another day. I hope that my story finds some kind of light for those of you that need it. Don't try and follow my path, try and learn from my path so maybe you don't have to endure some of the things that I have.

Remember that what you did for your country will always be a part of you. Don't let them take everything from you. Find a way to fit in and to go on and improve your life. Remember that this book was a look at me standing up and fighting for who I was, or for who I became. Maybe my struggles and actions can help someone else. Maybe this book will scream to them that they do matter, and no matter how hard they find it to fit in with society, or work you have to be strong and take that first step, and don't give up.

You are not alone.

You do have a choice.

If you feel you are at the end of your rope

If you feel you can't make it another minute,

I urge you to call 911.

Find whatever reason there is to make it to another day.

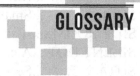

4187..................Army Personnel Action Formh
AA.....................Assembly area
AK.....................7.62 assault rifle
ANCOC.............Advanced Non-Commissioned Officer Course
BN.....................Battalion
BNCOC.............Basic Non-Commissioned Officer Course
CHALK.............Order of loading up military personnel
CONNEX..........Metal shipping container.
CSM ....Command Sergeant Major
C130.................U.S. Transport plane
DMV ....Department of motor vehicles
DZ ....Drop Zone
EEOC ....Equal Employment Opportunity Commission
FOB..................Forward operation base
HUMVEE ....Military vehicle
IED...................Improvised exploding device
LPN..................Licensed Practicing Nurse
LWOP...............Leave Without Pay
MD ....Medical Doctor
MSG.................Master Sergeant
M2 ....50 caliber machine gun
M4 ....version of m16 with a shorter barrel
NCO ....Non-Commissioned Officer
NCOIC ....Non-Commissioned Officer In Charge
NCOES ....Non-Commissioned Officer Education System
NOD.................Night Operating Device
OPSEC ....Operation Security
PCS ....Permanent Change of Station.
PMCS...............Preventive Measures Crisis Situation
PTSD................Post Traumatic Stress Disorder
PLF...................Parachutes Landing Fall
RED DOT ....Emergency alarm where assistance is needed immediately

RPG...................Rifle Propelled Grenade
SGLI..................Small Group Leadership Instructor
SIDE ROOM.....A small time out room with padded walls and floor
SILENT DOT....A call for assistance before situation arises
SHTA ....Security Hospital Treatment Assistant
SRSHTA............Senior Security Hospital Treatment Assistant
SWAP ....Exchange of working shifts
S2 ....Intelligence section of military operations
WTF ....What The Fuck
W/C...................Workers Compensation

ACKNOWLEDGMENTS

- Webster's II Dictionary—Third Edition
  Houghton Mifflin Company
  Boston, New York
  Copyright @ 2005
  www.houghtonmifflinbooks.com
  222 Berleley Street, Boston MA 02116

- New York State
  Department of Civil Service
  Andrew M. Cuomo—Governor
  Jerry Boone—Commissioner, President of the Civil Service
  Commission
  http://www.cs.ny.gov

- News & Star
  Sympathy and Bereavement Verses
  Telephone 01228 612612
  Dalston Road or Bank Street, Carlisle
  http://www.myfamilyannouncements.co.uk/newsandstar/
  verses

- iUniverse LLC
  1663 liberty Drive
  Bloomington, IN 47403
  www.iuniverse.com